IVF:
All You
Need to
Know

Clare Goulty

Clare has over twenty years' experience working in various senior roles for a FTSE 100 company. Her business experience includes fashion buying, marketing, communications and magazine publishing.

Sue Bedford

Sue is a fully qualified, practising nutritional therapist with a science background. Her specialist areas include fertility, women's health, child nutrition and wellness.

IVF:
All You Need to Know

A step-by-step
guide by leading
fertility experts

Compiled and
edited by
**Clare Goulty and
Sue Bedford**

Published by Lagom,
an imprint of Bonnier Books UK,
The Plaza,
535 Kings Road,
Chelsea Harbour,
London SW10 0SZ

www.bonnierbooks.co.uk

First published in paperback by Lagom in 2020

Paperback ISBN: 978-1-78606-947-4
Ebook ISBN: 978-1-78946-178-7

British Library Cataloguing-in-Publication Data:

A catalogue record for this book is available from the British Library.

Design by www.envydesign.co.uk

Printed and bound in Great Britain by Clays Ltd, Elcograf S.p.A

1 3 5 7 9 10 8 6 4 2

Selection, compilation and editing copyright © Clare Goulty and
Susan Bedford 2020
Copyright for individual contributors is stated at the end of each chapter

The right of the editors and compilers, and of the individual chapter authors, to be identified as the authors of this work has been asserted by them in accordance with the Copyright, Designs and Patents Act 1988.

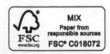

In dedication to
My inspirational parents, Rayella and Philip, who
always encouraged me to follow my dreams.
My wonderful husband, Brett, who supported me every
step of the way on our IVF journey.
My beautiful children, Sienna and Joshua – you are
my joy and will for ever be my most cherished life
achievement.
CLARE

In dedication to
My husband, Richard, and my three fab children,
Sophie, William and Lucy, for their ongoing support
with all of my nutrition ventures so far.
SUE

Contents

Acknowledgements

We would like to thank all of our expert contributors for their hard work and commitment. By contributing their industry-leading expertise they have enabled us to produce a comprehensive guide to IVF, of which we're most proud.

Many thanks to Sonia Land of Sheil Land Associates for helping us navigate the world of publishing. We really appreciate her guidance and expertise.

We're very grateful to our editor, Toby Buchan of Bonnier Books UK, for his superb editorial support and expert eye for detail.

Big thanks to the team at Lagom (Bonnier Books UK) for their marketing brilliance and enthusiasm for our book.

And heartfelt thanks to our readers. Wherever you currently are on your IVF journeys, we sincerely hope this guide brings you support and inspiration.

Introduction

1. IVF – we've done it, we created our beautiful families and we want you to succeed too!

Firstly, let us assure you that we've 'been there'. We've both travelled the challenging road of fertility treatment and have met and worked with leading IVF consultants in the UK and abroad.

2. We've met world-leading specialists along the way

Multiple cycles of IVF with leading fertility clinics in both the UK and abroad have introduced us to many world-leading IVF specialists. From our combined address book, we've invited some of those specialists to contribute chapters on their fields of expertise. This guide is a summary of their professional knowledge and experience.

3. Let us share with you their expertise

This book is a complete, specialist guide to IVF. It will take you through the entire IVF journey from explanation of treatment cycles to selecting a fertility clinic.

Questions such as how to optimise nutrition, how to prepare yourself emotionally and psychologically for IVF and whether sperm and egg quality can be potentially improved are considered.

Whilst neither of us took the egg- or sperm-donor route, we recognise that for some individuals/couples, the donor route is their best or only chance for IVF success. We've therefore included information on donor-assisted IVF.

Egg freezing is a growing trend, especially among career women who are delaying motherhood and also those with medical conditions who are looking for ways to preserve their fertility. We have therefore included information about the egg-freezing process and how to select a fertility clinic.

A section on real-life stories provides insight into a variety of different fertility journeys.

4. This guide is for you if . . .

This guide is for couples and individuals who are considering IVF and want to find out what's involved. It's also for those who may have already tried IVF but with no success. Often once couples and individuals complete their first cycle of IVF, they have a desire to learn more about the process and to discover ways to improve their chances of success next time around. And, as mentioned above, this guide includes information for those who may find themselves in the situation where their best chance of achieving a family is through donor-assisted IVF.

5. This guide was born because . . .

We decided to compile this guide because, in short, a specialist guide like this didn't exist when we were undertaking IVF. We wish it had. There's an abundance of information on IVF out there but it's often confusing and conflicting. Having met a broad group of leading IVF experts, we wanted to bring all of that expertise and knowledge together in one expert, comprehensive guide. When couples or individuals face IVF (either for the first time or multiple cycles), we feel it's important for them to be able to access a single source of expert, trusted and balanced information on IVF and the process.

6. About us:

Clare Goulty BA (hons), MBS, MBA

Clare has over twenty years' experience working in various senior roles for a FTSE 100 company. Her business experience includes fashion buying, marketing, communications and magazine publishing.

Sue Bedford BSc (Hons), PGCE, MSc, mBANT, CNHC

Sue is a fully qualified, practising nutritional therapist with a science background. Her specialist areas include fertility, women's health, child nutrition and wellbeing.

7. Meet our expert contributors:

Sally Cheshire, CBE, Chair of the Human Fertilisation and Embryology Authority (HFEA)

Sally, a former fertility patient herself, is Chair of the HFEA, the UK's regulator of the fertility sector and embryo research. She has held a number of senior leadership roles across the NHS and the wider health sector, and is currently also the Chair of Health Education England (North), which is responsible for the education and training of the 350,000 health and care staff across the North of England.

Sally previously enjoyed a successful corporate career with Deloitte, one of the global professional services firms and, having moved into public-sector work, is passionate about improving the quality of public services offered to patients and families across health and social care.

Professor Tim Child, MA, MD, MRCOG Medical Director, Oxford Fertility, Director, The Fertility Partnership, Associate Professor, University of Oxford

Tim Child is a prominent specialist in reproductive medicine, world renowned as the leader of the team that undertook the UK's first successful in vitro maturation (IVM) cycle resulting in the birth of twins in 2007. He is also the co-author of the UK's biggest-selling undergraduate textbook in obstetrics and gynaecology (Impey and Child; *Obstetrics and Gynaecology*). In 2004, he brought his expertise to the Oxford Fertility Clinic. His particular areas of interest are IVF, oocyte IVM, recurrent miscarriage, PCOS, reproductive immunology and laparoscopic surgery with special interest in endometriosis.

Mrs Mollie Graneek, independent psychotherapist and specialist fertility counsellor

Mollie Graneek began her career as a midwife and became concerned about the lack of emotional support for women struggling with sexual and reproductive health. She has continued to work in this field for the last forty-five years.

As a psychodynamic counsellor and Gestalt psychotherapist, Mollie skilfully integrates her clinical experience with the emotional support needed in the field of reproductive health issues. She works as a specialist fertility counsellor, with a particular interest in assisted reproduction and donor conception. She is also an accomplished writer and lecturer in this field.

She is accredited and registered as an independent psychotherapist and counsellor by British Association of Counsellors and Psychotherapists and United Kingdom Register of Counsellors.

Mollie became an executive member of the British

Infertility Counselling Association (BICA) and was appointed Chair in 2006. In the past she sat on the executive board of the British Society of Psychosomatic Obstetrics Gynaecology and Andrology (BSPOGA) and became its treasurer. She now spends her time working with different fertility clinics in London, offering support and advice to women or couples undergoing fertility treatment and gamete donation.

Christine Leary, BSc, HCPC, FRCPath, PhD

Christine is a consultant embryologist and director at the Hull IVF Unit, with more than fifteen years' experience. She is responsible for managing the Embryology Laboratory and Quality Management. In 2013, she became a Fellow of the Royal College of Pathologists and she has recently completed a doctoral thesis on the effects of maternal weight and obesity on the viability and metabolism of human oocytes and embryos.

Christine currently holds a number of additional positions and is a teaching fellow at the Hull York Medical School, an Executive Committee member of the British Fertility Society, and a Professional Development Committee member for the Association of Clinical Embryologists.

INTRODUCTION

Alison Leverett-Morris, MA, BA (Hons), ADHP, NSHP&M, UKCP

Alison Leverett-Morris is an integrative hypno-psychotherapist, specialising in fertility and mind-body health. Alison runs Fertile Mind and Body, a private practice offering therapeutic services (in person and online) to optimise fertility and support individuals and couples at every stage of their fertility journey.

Alison's specialisation in fertility developed further to her personal experience of having fertility treatment over a ten-year period. Recognising the complexity and impact of fertility issues, Alison offers a holistic mind-body approach to fertility, which complements assisted reproductive techniques such as IVF. Alison's practice is informed by clinical evidence of how mind-body approaches such as hypnotherapy can enhance fertility and increase pregnancy outcome. Alison is a fully accredited member of the UK Council of Psychotherapy (UKCP) and trains therapists for the National College of Hypnosis and Psychotherapy. She can be contacted at www.alisonleverettmorris.co.uk and www.fertilemindandbody.co.uk.

Tracey Sainsbury, lead fertility counsellor at the London Women's Clinic

Tracey is a specialist accredited fertility counsellor with over twenty years' experience working and volunteering in the field of infertility. She initially volunteered, and later worked with iSSUE and Child, the two charities that merged to form Infertility Network UK in 2003, now called the Fertility Network. Since 2011, Tracey has worked as a counsellor providing support and implications counselling in leading London clinics and egg banks including the London Women's Clinic, the Bridge Centre, London Egg Bank, London Sperm Bank and the Lister Fertility Clinic.

Tracey has been a member of the British Infertility Counselling Association (BICA) Executive Committee, having previously represented the voice of the patient on the BICA Accreditation Board. She was a member of the National Donation Strategy Group and Lifecycle Editorial Board set up by the HFEA to promote best practice for gamete donors, sits on the Steering Group for Fertility Fest, and remains a counselling member of the Advisory Panel for Fertility Network and a Trustee for the Sperm Egg and Embryo Donation Trust (SEED Trust).

Neema Savvides, BSc (Hons), DipNT, mBANT

Based at the Harley Street Fertility Clinic, Neema specialises in male and female fertility and women's health. She is passionate about nutrition, its impact on the body, how it makes you feel, and in turn how it can affect an individual's fertility. She is a nutritional therapist who helps to support couples who are preparing for and experiencing IVF.

Laura Spoelstra, previously chief executive of the National Gamete Donation Trust (now known as the SEED Trust)

Laura Spoelstra gave birth to twins in 1998. Shortly afterwards, she responded to a call for altruistic egg donors and donated at a UK clinic. In 2003, she joined the National Gamete Donation Trust (NGDT), becoming chair in 2004 and chief executive from 2012–16. This national organisation is now called SEED Trust (Sperm Egg and Embryo Donation Trust). Laura continues to contribute to media discussions about egg and sperm donation.

CHAPTER 1

Selecting a Fertility Clinic and What to Expect

Sally Cheshire CBE, Chair of the Human Fertilisation
and Embryology Authority (HFEA)

1. Introduction

I am delighted that we have been asked to contribute a chapter to this book to help you make the best possible choice about where to have your treatment.

The HFEA is the UK's independent regulator overseeing fertility treatment and research. We make sure clinics offer a safe, effective and lawful service. We also provide clear and impartial information – free of charge – to everyone affected by assisted reproduction. We know that choosing the right clinic is one of the most important decisions you'll make. After all, you're relying on them to give you the best possible chance of having a baby and to support you through one of life's toughest challenges.

We know from talking to patients that you want to base

the decisions about your treatment and where to have it on more than just success rates. Of course you want to maximise your chances of getting pregnant, but you also want to know that the clinic is well run and offers a caring service. We can give you this information and I will talk about how to interpret that in this chapter.

I've been a fertility patient, so I know how tough this process is and how confusing it can all feel. With our experience, knowledge and oversight of all the fertility clinics in the UK, we can hopefully help you feel more confident about the decisions that lie ahead.

2. Selecting a fertility clinic

There are around 120 fertility clinics in the UK, from small ones specialising in certain treatments to large clinics performing thousands of cycles a year. In this chapter we'll explore what makes a good clinic, how to prepare for your first appointment and what kind of decisions you'll need to make during your treatment.

3. Starting the process

If you've been trying to have a family for some time, there's sometimes a temptation to get on with treatment as soon as possible. However, it's really worth taking some time to understand your diagnosis, learn about the different treatments and add-ons to your treatment that the clinic might offer you, and research the right clinic.

The more informed you are, the easier it will be to make key decisions throughout your treatment and the more in control you'll feel at every stage of the process. This is a complicated field, but with a little preparation and research you'll be able to start your fertility journey in the best possible way: being as prepared as you can be for what's round the corner.

There's so much with fertility that we can't control, that being on top of the decisions we can make is all the more important. Take your time, talk to as many people as possible and don't be afraid to ask questions. Fertility treatment may be an emotional rollercoaster, but that doesn't mean you can't gauge what's in store before you get on board.

4. What to look for when choosing a clinic

Whether your treatment is funded by the NHS, or you're paying for it yourself, you'll want to make sure it's the right clinic for you. Some clinics cater for self-funding and NHS patients and with so many to choose from, deciding which one best meets your needs can feel a bit overwhelming.

Some of the factors you may wish to consider when choosing a clinic include:

Treatments offered
- Eligibility criteria
- Cost

- Location — bear in mind you'll probably need to make multiple trips to your clinic, sometimes at short notice

- How other patients have rated the clinic on our Choose a Fertility Clinic service

- How HFEA inspectors have rated the clinic

- The clinic's birth and multiple birth rates

- Waiting times for donor eggs or sperm (if applicable)

- Convenience and availability of counselling provision

Much of this information is available on the HFEA website (www.hfea.gov.uk), so that's a good place to start browsing to help you narrow down your options. In some cases, if you're looking to have a slightly less common treatment or you're over a certain age the number of clinics available to you may be more limited.

5. NHS or private funding

One of the first decisions you'll want to consider is whether to try to have IVF through the NHS or pay for it yourself. The rules around NHS funding are complicated, so the best thing to do is to talk to your GP about what is available and whether you are eligible for treatment.

Broadly speaking, England, Wales, Scotland and

Northern Ireland all make their own decisions about funding IVF treatment, which means they may have different eligibility criteria and fund different numbers of cycles. Within England it gets more complicated as decisions around funding fertility treatment are made at a local level by Clinical Commissioning Groups (CCGs) – a group of people with expertise in buying health services who make decisions about which treatments to provide in their area. This means that depending on where you live you may be able to get three, two, one or (rarely) no IVF cycles at all. In addition, you may not be able to choose your own clinic if your local CCG has a contract with a particular provider. Talk to your GP to find out what's available in your area and what the rules are around choosing your clinic.

Alternatively, you can choose to pay for fertility treatment yourself. Private costs for fertility treatment are not regulated, which means that prices can vary considerably. In some cases, the same treatment can be two or even three times more expensive depending on which clinic you go to, so it's definitely worth exploring the different centre options if you can. When you're comparing prices make sure that you're comparing like for like. Some clinics will quote for the treatment only – IVF or Intracytoplasmic sperm injection (ICSI), a treatment that only differs from IVF in that instead of mixing the sperm with the eggs and leaving them to fertilise, an embryologist will inject a single sperm into the egg – but not include any essential extras, such as an initial consultation, health tests or medication, which are typically hundreds or thousands of pounds. When you're getting quotes, ask for a fully costed personalised treatment plan that details all of the essential costs, with any optional extras listed separately. Depending on the treatment you're having and which clinic you choose, you may need to pay for the following in addition to your basic treatment:

- An initial consultation
- Further consultations or assessments
- Health tests/infection screening
- Fertility drugs
- Sperm analysis
- Freezing and storing leftover embryos
- Transferring frozen embryos

During treatment, costs can sometimes increase above the original estimate; therefore don't treat your quote as set in stone. It might be that you need further tests or treatments that the clinic hadn't originally anticipated, so it's always a good idea to have a contingency fund available.

Depending on the clinic you choose, you may also be offered treatment add-ons on top of your regular IVF or ICSI at an additional cost. Many of these are emerging treatments with some promising, limited results but no concrete evidence that they improve pregnancy rates. Some of them have no evidence at all. Prices for treatment add-ons can run into the thousands of pounds, potentially doubling your final bill for treatment. It's crucial to be informed about the add-ons that may be offered, so that you can ask the right questions, and make the right choices, when choosing what treatment to have. At the HFEA, we've produced 'traffic light' rated information on our website that keeps up-to-date with the latest evidence on each of the most commonly offered add-ons.

If cost is an issue for you, you may be offered the chance of joining an egg-sharing programme. Egg sharing is when a woman who is already having fertility treatment donates some of her eggs to the clinic where she's having treatment for use by other women who can't use their own eggs. Usually if you share your eggs your clinic will offer you free or discounted treatment, although bear in mind you'll still need to meet the same eligibility criteria as egg donors, so it's not available to everyone.

Choosing to share your eggs is a serious decision, which is why your clinic will offer you counselling before you make a final decision. This is to help you think through all the issues involved in egg sharing, such as how you'll feel if the woman you donated your eggs to gets pregnant and you don't. You also need to think through how you would feel about being contacted by any children born from your donation when they reach eighteen and how your child might feel about having donor half-siblings. Not all clinics offer egg sharing, so you'll need to find one that does.

6. Eligibility for treatment

There are no age limits for fertility treatment in UK law, so the decision on whether someone of a certain age can be treated is down to their clinic. Clinicians need to decide whether a patient's health will allow them to go through treatment and a possible pregnancy and weigh up any potential health risks against their chance of conceiving through IVF. The HFEA also requires clinics to carry out a 'Welfare of the Child' assessment before starting any treatment. This looks at factors that are likely to cause serious physical, psychological or medical harm, either to the child to be born or to any existing child of the family.

Some clinics have additional criteria such as a body mass index (BMI) within a certain range, while others only treat private patients. Contact your shortlist of possible clinics to find out if you are eligible for treatment there.

7. Understanding the data

For many people, a clinic's success rates are one of the most important factors they consider when choosing a clinic. The HFEA collects statistics on the outcome of every treatment a clinic performs and publishes these through its 'Choose a Fertility Clinic' tool on its website. Although clinics often publish their own success rates, we always recommend you access the data on our website to ensure you're comparing like with like.

On www.hfea.gov.uk you can view:

- IVF birth rates for women up to the age of thirty-eight and those of thirty-eight-plus, both from one treatment and from a full cycle

- Donor insemination birth rates for women up to the age of thirty-eight, and those of thirty-eight-plus

- The number of cycles the clinic has performed

- How the clinic compares to the national average

- Multiple birth rates

How reliable the data is depends upon how many treatment cycles the clinic has performed. Generally, the more cycles, the more confident we are that the data is an accurate reflection of their success rate. This shouldn't deter you from smaller clinics, however, as many of them offer more specialist treatments or have experience treating certain kinds of patients, which may be relevant to your situation.

It's understandable that many people will focus exclusively on success rates when comparing clinics. Try not to do this! Although they may have slightly different success rates, the majority of clinics are just as good as each other and your chance of getting pregnant at each one is about the same for you as an individual or as a couple. That's why it's important to focus on whether the clinic's rates are comparable to the national average and, more importantly, how the clinic meets your needs.

Also, differences of just one or two percentage points are often down to chance rather than being a reflection of a clinic's abilities: a clinic that's performing particularly well one year may have lower success rates the following year and vice versa. In these cases, if you're comparing two or more clinics you may want to consider the multiple other variables (cost, location, patient ratings) to find a clinic that meets all your needs and expectations rather than deciding on success rates alone.

The HFEA also publishes success rates per egg collection. This shows how many women get pregnant in a particular clinic after all their embryos from one egg collection have been used, regardless of how many different embryo transfers she has. This gives a much better picture of success as most women need more than one transfer to get pregnant. It's understandable to think, 'If I have a one in three chance of getting pregnant then I should get pregnant after the third cycle.' But that's not how it works: your chance is the same each time, but over multiple transfers, the overall chance of success increases gradually.

8. You're not a success rate

It's easy to see success rates and immediately apply them to ourselves. However, success rates give an indication of the clinic's performance overall; they don't give you your individual prognosis. Every woman and couple is different and a lot depends on how long you have been trying and how your embryos appear once created in the laboratory. Even if you know other people who are in a similar position to you and they're successful, there's no guarantee you will be too. Talk to your doctor about your individual chances of success and treat the statistics as a broad indication of the success of different treatments rather than as a tool for predicting your own outcome.

9. Multiple births

A multiple birth (twins, triplets or more) is the single greatest health risk to both mum and babies.

Some of the risks to mums of multiple births include:

- A higher risk of early or late miscarriages.
- An increased risk of high blood pressure – 20 per cent of mothers of twins suffer from high blood pressure (hypertension), compared to only 1 to 5 per cent of mothers of single babies.
- An increased risk of the mother developing pre-eclampsia - up to 30 per cent for twin pregnancies compared to 2 to 10 per cent in single-baby pregnancies.
- An increased risk of problems such as haemorrhage and anaemia.
- The risk of the mother dying is twice as high during twin pregnancy or birth.

- New mothers may be more vulnerable to mental health problems like stress and depression.

Some of the risks to the babies include:

- Between 40 and 60 per cent of IVF twins need to be transferred to the neonatal care unit when they are born. By comparison, only 20 per cent of single IVF babies need the same level of care.

- 8 per cent of twins need help with their breathing and 6 per cent suffer from respiratory distress syndrome (breathing difficulties) compared with 1.5 per cent and 0.8 per cent for single babies.

- The risk of death around the time of birth is three to six times higher for twins and nine times higher for triplets. A study from 2003 estimated that if all IVF babies born in the UK had been single babies, the deaths of 126 babies could have been avoided.

- A small percentage of twins have severe health problems that will affect their entire lives (for example cerebral palsy, which affects between four and six times as many twins compared with singleton babies).

- Prematurity and low birth weight carry the risk of lower IQ and are linked with Attention Deficit Hyperactivity Disorder (ADHD) and long-lasting behavioural difficulties.

The risk of a multiple birth can be reduced by transferring only one embryo to the womb (elective single embryo transfer or eSET) rather than two or three, which used to be the norm. Success rates are broadly the same or higher for eSETs and you're much less likely to have a multiple pregnancy, with all the risks that come with that.

Because of these health risks the HFEA has implemented a policy which has lowered the multiple birth rate to around 10 per cent of IVF births which means clinics should be giving eSETs to patients wherever possible. Many clinics have made excellent progress towards this target without lowering success rates. When looking for a clinic you should look for one with a low multiple-birth rate but a high success rate to maximise your chance of having a safe and healthy pregnancy.

Headline birth rates take multiple pregnancy into account, so a clinic with a high birth rate and low multiple birth rate will come out higher than one with a high birth rate and a high multiple rate.

10. Learning from others

10.1 Patient ratings
While we can easily compare hard facts like costs, success rates and treatments offered; it's much harder to get a sense of what it would really be like to be treated at a particular clinic. Everything from how caring the staff are to how easily you can book or amend an appointment can

contribute to a good (or bad) experience. This is especially important with fertility treatment, as it's already such a physically and emotionally demanding time that the last thing you want is to be worrying about your clinic.

Talking to others about their experience of a clinic can give you an indication of how well a clinic is meeting its patients' needs. To encourage this kind of information sharing we ask people who've had fertility treatment to rate their clinic in five areas:

1. How likely are you to recommend this clinic to friends and family if they needed similar care or treatment?

2. To what extent did you feel you understood everything that was happening throughout your treatment?

3. Did you pay what you expected?

4. To what extent did you feel you were treated with privacy and dignity?

5. How was the level of empathy and understanding shown towards you by the clinic team?

You can see the results by searching for any licensed clinic on our website.

You may also find it helpful to visit the clinic before you've committed to having treatment there to meet the staff and get a feel for the facilities and environment. If there are other patients there you could ask them how they've found the clinic and whether they would recommend it.

Online forums such as www.fertilityfriends.co.uk and www.fertilitynetworkuk.org are good places to ask for clinic recommendations in your area, or for feedback on a particular clinic.

10.2 Inspection ratings

Part of the HFEA's role as a regulator is to inspect clinics every two years against a number of important standards that, as a patient, may not be at the forefront of your mind when you're researching clinics. These include whether the clinic stores patients' eggs, sperm and embryos safely, whether they have the appropriate equipment and facilities to deliver safe, effective treatment and whether they have suitably qualified staff.

These are all essential components of a good clinic but aren't things you can necessarily determine yourself. To help you to make an informed decision therefore, we publish an inspection report on every clinic and indicate a 'star rating' which corresponds to the length of licence (in years) we have issued.

We also highlight clinics where we have serious concerns about their performance. These clinics are inspected on a more frequent basis and if they don't improve quickly enough, or we have serious concerns that their activities may be causing harm to patients, their sperm, eggs or embryos we will consider removing their licence. Thankfully, most clinics respond well and the HFEA rarely considers removing licences.

You can see the inspection ratings by searching for any licensed clinic on the HFEA website: www.hfea.gov.uk. You can also read inspection reports, which are detailed assessments of how a clinic is performing.

11. What makes a good clinic?

- Success rates that are consistent with or higher than the national average
- A multiple birth rate that's consistent with or lower than the national average
- Good patient ratings
- Good inspection ratings
- A comprehensive counselling service

12. Counselling

Many women and men say that going through fertility treatment was one of the hardest things they've ever had to do. Being confronted with family, friends or colleagues who are starting their families can be a painful reminder of your own difficulties, even when you're happy for their good fortune. Counselling can help you to handle those feelings as well as coping with any disappointments you may suffer on the way. It's not a sign that you're ill or unable to cope. Counselling is as essential as any other component of your treatment and should be a key factor you consider when choosing a clinic.

Although every licensed UK clinic is required to offer you counselling, how they practically deliver on that commitment can vary. Some clinics may have a counsellor available on-site so you can talk to them whenever you need, while others might refer you to a counsellor who's only available at certain times during the week; others offer Skype or phone consultations. Talk to your clinic to find out how their counselling service works and whether there are any limits on how frequently you can access support. A good clinic is one that understands the difficult emotional situation you're facing and takes as much care with your emotional wellbeing as with your physical health.

13. Making your decision

One of the benefits of having treatment at a licensed clinic in the UK is that the HFEA has a strong and effective regulatory system to protect patients, their embryos, eggs and sperm. We inspect clinics at least every two years to ensure they're maintaining high standards and we have enforcement powers at our disposal if we're concerned a clinic isn't improving fast enough.

Hopefully the information we've provided will help you choose the clinic that is best suited to your needs and will give you the best possible chance of having the family you want. But no matter which clinic you choose you can have confidence that if it's licensed, it's meeting key quality and safety standards. This should reassure you and be one less thing to worry about.

You can search for a licensed clinic using the 'Choose a Fertility Clinic tool' on the HFEA website.

14. Preparing for your first clinic appointment

It's natural to feel a bit apprehensive before attending your first clinic appointment. Remember that your clinic wants you to be successful as much as you do and they should have your best interests at heart. They'll have supported many women and men through the same process you're going through and will hopefully understand how daunting and new this whole experience is for you.

At the clinic, don't be afraid to ask as many questions as you need to. You are paying for a service and it's the clinic's responsibility to ensure you understand and are comfortable with everything that's happening. You should also take your time to think through any decisions that need to be made, and get advice or support from alternative sources if you need to. Never feel pressured to rush into a decision that you're not 100 per cent happy with.

Some questions you might want to ask at the clinic include:

- What are the benefits of the treatment you've recommended and why do you think it's the best option for me?

- How many patients at your clinic have had this treatment in the last two years, and how many of them have become pregnant/had a baby?

- Are there alternative treatments? If so, what do they involve, and why do you think they are less suitable for me?

- What other options are available to me if this treatment doesn't work?

- How does my age affect the choice of fertility treatment?

- What drugs will I have to take and what are the usual side effects they might have?

- Are there any alternatives to the drugs you have mentioned?

- Can you break down all the costs involved in this treatment? Are there any other costs that might arise? (Your clinic should provide you with a costed treatment plan.)

- Is there any way these costs can be reduced?

- What lifestyle changes can I make to boost my chance of success (e.g. diet, exercise, stopping smoking, etc.)? How will these help?

- What kind of counselling or advice service do you provide? Is there a cost for this, or how many free sessions can I have?

- Does this clinic have a patient support group I can join, or are there other groups you would recommend?

- Could you tell me more about the assessment process you will need to carry out before giving me the go-ahead for treatment (this is sometimes known as the 'welfare of the child' assessment)?

- What happens next? Do I (and/or my partner) need to do anything now?

15. What to expect at the clinic

When you start treatment at a clinic, what happens next will depend on your circumstances. In many cases you'll start treatment straight away but in others you may be given further fertility tests if your existing tests haven't identified the cause of infertility. These tests can include:

15.1 For women

- A full hormone profile taken between days two and four of your period to assess for any hormone imbalance.

- Blood tests to find out if you are ovulating.

- An ultrasound scan to look at your uterus and ovaries.

- Follicle tracking — a series of ultrasound scans to follow the development of a follicle to see if an egg is developing.

- Hysterosalpingogram – an X-ray to check your fallopian tubes.

- Laparoscopy – an operation in which a dye is injected through your cervix as the pelvis is inspected via a telescope (laparoscope) with a tiny camera attached to check for tubal blockage.

- Hysteroscopy – a telescope with a camera attached is used to view your uterus to check for conditions such as fibroids or polyps.

- Hysterosalpingo-contrast sonography (HyCoSy) – a vaginal ultrasound probe is used to check the fallopian tubes for blockages.

- Occasionally, a tissue sample may be taken from the endometrium lining of your uterus to be analysed.

15.2 For men

- Semen analysis to check sperm numbers and quality.

- Sperm antibody test to check for protein molecules. that may prevent sperm from fertilising an egg.

In 25 per cent of cases the cause of infertility is unknown, which can make it difficult for clinics to choose the most appropriate treatment. It can understandably be frustrating not knowing what the problem is and how to fix it, but sadly fertility treatment isn't an exact science. How you handle this is up to you: some people prefer to let their consultant make decisions in their best interests, while others like to do as much research as possible into their situation so they can make decisions about how to move forward jointly with their treating clinician.

16. Health checks

Before having treatment, everyone involved is required to have health checks to prevent certain serious conditions from being passed on to the mother or child. You'll be tested for:

- HIV 1 and 2 (Anti-HIV – 1, 2)

- Hepatitis B: (HBsAg/Anti-HBc)

- Hepatitis C: (Anti-HCV-Ab)

If you've travelled recently you may also be tested for infectious diseases such as malaria, so make sure you let your clinic know about any recent trips abroad.

If you have a serious genetic condition in your family, it may be possible for you to have a treatment called pre-implantation genetic diagnosis (PGD), which tests the embryos to see if any of them are affected by the condition. Only those that are unaffected are transferred to the womb, which will not only protect your future child but remove the chance of the condition being passed on through your family.

You should discuss any genetic conditions in your family

with your clinic and they can advise on an appropriate course of action. To find out more about PGD, go to the HFEA website.

17. Giving consent to treatment

Before you can start treatment, you'll need to complete a number of consent forms. This isn't just paperwork; it's an important opportunity to ensure your sperm, eggs, embryos and personal information are used in a way that you're happy with. You should take the time to understand exactly what you're giving consent to and that you've thought through all the implications. The forms you may need to complete include:

17.1 Consent to your fertility treatment

This is similar to the form you have to sign for many other medical treatments and essentially allows your clinic to give you your agreed treatment. It's important that before you sign the form your clinic has clearly explained to you what your treatment involves and that you are entitled to receive counselling.

17.2 Consent to disclosure of information by your clinic

Your clinic is not allowed to tell your GP or anyone else about your treatment unless they have your consent to do so. Most patients are happy for other clinical staff, like their GP or midwife, to know about their fertility treatment but others prefer to keep it confidential. Clinics also need your permission to allow auditors and finance staff to see your records.

17.3 Consent to disclosure of information by the HFEA

Clinics collect treatment information, some of which is provided to the HFEA and held securely by us. We're able to use this data to publish clinic success rates on our website and to study trends in fertility treatment, which helps to inform clinics, researchers and the wider public. Occasionally, researchers ask us for patient-identifying information to help with their research projects but we can only provide that data if you've consented for us to do so. These researchers might link fertility patients' information to other health databases, to see if fertility treatment has any link with diseases like cancer or birth defects (the research so far is showing very reassuring results). Only research projects that meet strict guidelines are allowed to access personal information that would identify individual patients. You can find out more about the information we collect and about the disclosure of personal information to researchers on the HFEA website.

17.4 Consent to the use and storage of sperm, eggs and/or any embryos produced from them

You'll need to consent to your eggs, sperm or embryos

being used for your own treatment, the treatment of others or for research, or for training purposes. If you freeze any of your sperm, eggs or embryos you'll need to make clear how long they should be frozen for and the conditions under which they can be used.

Your clinic will also ask you to think about what should happen to any frozen embryos if you or your partner were to die or become unable to make decisions. These are tough issues to consider but it's very important you've thought them through carefully just in case something unexpected happens.

17.5 Consent to parenthood

If you're having treatment with donated sperm, eggs or embryos and you're not married or in a civil partnership, you and your partner will need to sign the relevant consent forms to ensure that your partner is recognised as the child's legal parent. If this form isn't completed properly there's a risk that your partner won't be recognised as the child's legal parent and they'll need to go through a lengthy court process to adopt their child.

17.6 Withdrawing consent

It is possible for you to withdraw your consent providing your eggs, sperm and embryos haven't already been used in treatment, research or training (depending on what you consented to). Your partner or donor can also change or withdraw their consent at any time until their eggs, sperm or embryos have been used in treatment. If that happens you wouldn't be able to continue with treatment, even if the embryos have been jointly created with your eggs or sperm. This may be a rare occurrence but it is something you need to consider.

Once you've had any necessary health testing, have completed your health checks and signed all the relevant consent forms, you should be ready to start your treatment.

18. Decisions during treatment

There are certain decisions you'll need to make during your treatment to ensure any embryos you create are used in ways you're happy with.

18.1 Embryo transfer

In the past, most women had two or more embryos transferred to their womb. However, we now know that this considerably increases your chance of having a multiple birth (twins, triplets or more), which poses serious risks to the health of both mum and babies (as already discussed on pages 11–13). It is now normal for most women to have only one embryo transferred (eSET) and any remaining embryos frozen. This has no impact on success rates and is considerably safer for the mother and embryos. Not everyone is eligible for eSET though, so you should talk to your clinician about whether it's right for you.

18.2 Storing your embryos

Any embryos that you don't use in your first treatment cycle will need to be frozen and stored. On your consent-to-storage form (see above) you'll be asked to decide how long you'd like your embryos to be stored for. The maximum storage period for embryos in the UK is ten years except for women who, for medical reasons, are eligible for an extension of up to fifty-five years. Your clinic will be able to explain if this applies to you.

It's very important that you let your clinic know if you change address. This is particularly true if you have decided to store your embryos for less than ten years because if the clinic can't reach you they may have to take your embryos out of storage and allow them to perish.

If you have the option to store for fifty-five years, you'll need to confirm every ten years that you want to continue storing your embryos and your doctor will need to confirm that you're eligible to do so. Again, it's vital that you stay in touch with your clinic to prevent your embryos from being discarded if your storage runs out. (See Chapter 6 for more details.)

19. What to do with leftover embryos

If you have leftover frozen embryos in storage, you'll need to consider what you'd like to do with them. Some people prefer to discard them, which involves removing them from the freezer and allowing them to perish naturally in warmer temperatures or water. If you'd rather your embryos weren't discarded, then you can donate them to someone else's treatment, fertility research or training.

If you'd like to donate them to someone else's treatment, it's important that you're aware of the implications of this. In the UK, we have identifiable donation, which means a child conceived with your donation can ask for your name, date of birth and contact details when they turn eighteen. You'll need to be prepared for the possibility that a child conceived with your donation may attempt to make contact with you at some point – and for the possibility that they won't.

Your other option is to donate any leftover embryos to research or training. Embryo research has the potential to develop new treatments for infertility and genetic diseases. For example, recent research has led to the development of ground-breaking treatment for people with severe mitochondrial disease. Mitochondrial disease is incurable, genetic and often fatal. Some children born with the disease never reach adulthood while others suffer from debilitating symptoms. Thanks to research, there now exists a treatment that can prevent mitochondrial disease from being passed on to a sufferer's children, thereby eradicating the disease from the next generation.

Alternatively, you can donate your embryos to support the training of the next generation of embryologists. Trainee embryologists need practice working with real embryos to help them master certain tricky and delicate techniques before they can provide treatment to patients.

To find out more about donating your embryos to somebody else's treatment, research or training, speak to your clinic.

20. After treatment

Once you've finished treatment at your clinic the HFEA would really appreciate it if you could give feedback by rating your clinic on our website. Your ratings are invaluable in helping other people decide if a clinic is right for them and helps to create an open and transparent market for fertility services where patients are equipped with the necessary information and your feedback to help them make the right choices. Your feedback encourages clinics to continue to improve their service to ensure their patients' satisfaction is reflected in their ratings. Search for your clinic on the HFEA website to give your ratings.

21. Making a complaint

Unfortunately, not everyone has the positive clinic experience they were hoping for. If you're not happy with your treatment you should follow your clinic's complaint process to see if they can set things straight. If the problem is not resolved to your satisfaction you may be able to refer the complaint to the HFEA.

22. Conclusion

In this chapter we've discussed some of the key issues you may want to think about before choosing a fertility clinic, including what to look for in a clinic, how to prepare for your clinic appointment and decisions you'll need to make during your treatment. Unlike many other medical treatments, you may be receiving fertility treatment from the same clinic for months or even years, so taking the time to make an informed decision now could have a big impact on your future wellbeing. A great clinic isn't just one that can give you effective treatment: it's one with compassionate staff, clear pricing structures, seamless administrative processes and exceptional emotional support. Finding a clinic that excels in all these areas could be of vital importance in the weeks and months to come.

Hopefully the information we've provided here will help make your decision that little bit easier, but if you need more information on fertility treatments and clinics there's a wealth of knowledge on our website: www.hfea. gov.uk.

CHAPTER 2

The IVF Process and Different Types of Treatment Cycles

Professor Tim Child MA, MD, MRCOG,
Medical Director, Oxford Fertility, Director,
The Fertility Partnership, Associate Professor,
University of Oxford

1. Introduction

In vitro fertilisation (IVF) is an established treatment for the devastating disease of infertility. Indeed, in most developed countries, including the UK, at least 1 per cent of babies born each year are conceived through IVF. While IVF was developed in the 1970s as a treatment for couples with infertility due to fallopian tube damage, it soon became apparent that the treatment could be similarly successful with other causes of infertility too, such as lack of ovulation, endometriosis or unexplained infertility. With the advent of the intracytoplasmic sperm injection (ICSI) in the 1990s, couples with severe male factor infertility (previously requiring donor sperm) were also able to access treatment, allowing them to have their own biological child.

The aim of this chapter is to review the procedures which make up 'assisted conception', including IVF, ICSI, egg and embryo freezing, blastocyst culture, embryo transfer, frozen embryo replacement, surgical sperm retrieval, biopsy and genetic analysis of embryos, and also newer 'add-on' techniques such as endometrial scratch and embryo glue. (A blastocyst is an embryo in an early stage of its development, usually 5-6 days after fertilisation.)

2. IVF

In a normal menstrual cycle one ovarian follicle, containing a single egg, develops each month and ovulates around mid-cycle. In an IVF cycle one egg is insufficient to achieve acceptable pregnancy rates, and so injected drugs, called gonadotropins (e.g. Gonal-F or Menopur), are used to stimulate the woman's ovaries to produce multiple follicles. Eggs are collected under sedation using a needle passed, via a vaginal ultrasound scan probe, into the ovarian follicles. On average five to fifteen eggs are retrieved, are inseminated with sperm, and then left overnight to fertilise. Around two thirds of eggs fertilise normally (and are now termed embryos) and are cultured in an incubator for two to six days until the best one or two are identified for transfer back to the womb (embryo transfer or 'ET'). Spare embryos of suitable quality are frozen for later use. A urine or blood pregnancy test is performed around sixteen days after the egg collection. If the test shows the woman to be pregnant, then a scan to confirm the viability and number of pregnancies is performed two to three weeks after the pregnancy test. At that point women are usually referred back to their GP for pregnancy care.

The drugs used to stimulate the ovaries are gonadotropins and contain follicle stimulating hormone (FSH). They are either derived from urine (such as Menopur) or recombinant (made in the laboratory, such as Gonal-F). Most experts think urinary and recombinant gonadotropins lead to similar IVF success rates. They are given by daily subcutaneous injection into the skin of the abdomen or thigh for ten to fourteen days. If gonadotropins are given alone they will drive the ovaries on to ever larger multiple follicles, leading to ovulation and loss of all of the eggs. Therefore, during an IVF cycle a second drug needs to be given to prevent ovulation. These drugs are either agonists, used as part of the long protocol, or antagonists, used in the short protocol.

In a long-protocol cycle, the agonists are often started on day 21 of the menstrual cycle. Most IVF centres use a daily low dose agonist given by subcutaneous injection or by nasal spray, taken for two to three weeks to achieve down-regulation of the pituitary gland in which all of the 'reproductive hormones' are switched off. Once down-regulation is confirmed, the gonadotropins are started alongside the continued daily agonist drug. As long as the agonist is continued the woman is very unlikely to ovulate. In a short-protocol cycle, gonadotropins are started first, on day 2 of menstruation, and then after five to seven days the antagonist is added and is given by daily subcutaneous injection. The antagonists are continued alongside the daily gonadotropin injection in order to prevent ovulation. In addition to being a shorter treatment, short-protocol antagonist cycles result in a significantly lower risk of the main complication of IVF, ovarian hyperstimulation syndrome (OHSS). There is some debate as to whether the success rate of short-protocol antagonist cycles is slightly lower than long-protocol treatments.

The dose of gonadotropin is chosen based on an assessment of the woman's ovarian reserve. The higher the ovarian reserve the greater the number of eggs resting in the ovaries and the lower the gonadotropin dose prescribed. Too high an ovarian response can lead to the development of OHSS. Ovarian reserve is usually assessed by blood tests (FSH and AMH) and ultrasound (antral follicle count – AFC). In addition, the age of the woman is considered (ovarian reserve falls with age) and the response to any previous ovarian stimulation.

The ovarian response to gonadotropin stimulation is assessed by ultrasound monitoring every few days plus, in most centres, blood tests for oestradiol levels. With a monitoring scan the sonographer measures the number and size of ovarian follicles. Based on this, and the oestradiol result, the doctor may decide to continue stimulation at the same gonadotropin dose or to increase or decrease the dose. A further monitoring scan may be arranged.

Once it is felt that there are an optimal number of mature size follicles (often considered to be 12–20mm diameter) then the decision is made to move on to the egg collection. A further drug needs to be given to switch on final maturation of the eggs. This is sometimes called the 'late night' or 'trigger' injection and mimics the LH (luteinising hormone) surge which naturally occurs in a menstrual cycle and which leads to ovulation. In an IVF cycle, LH can be given to switch on maturation but, more commonly, the biochemically similar hormone hCG is used as it lasts longer in the body and is associated with a higher IVF success rate. The ovaries would normally ovulate forty-eight hours or so after the 'trigger' hCG injection and the eggs would be lost. Therefore the woman is, instead, brought in for the oocyte collection procedure thirty-four to thirty-eight hours (depending on the clinic) after the trigger injection.

Egg collections are usually done under light sedation with a drug administered into a drip in the hand or arm. Sometimes a general anaesthetic is used (in which breathing is paralysed and so a ventilator is required). The woman's legs are placed in stirrups and a scan probe introduced into her vagina. The probe has a needle attached to it and, under scan guidance, the doctor pushes the tip of the needle through the vaginal skin into the first ovary. Once the needle tip is within a follicle the doctor uses a foot pedal to aspirate follicular fluid into a test tube (this is the only time the eggs are in a test-tube, despite the commonly used term 'test-tube baby'). The test tubes are passed to an embryologist who pours the fluid into a Petri dish to examine, using a microscope, for eggs. The egg collection procedure takes around 20 minutes. If a fresh sample from the male partner is being used he will be asked to produce around the same time. If donor sperm is used it will be thawed.

The sperm sample is then prepared in the laboratory. If the sperm function is normal (normal count, motility, volume, and percentage of normal forms) then conventional IVF is used in which around 100,000 motile sperm are added to each egg to inseminate them. If the sperm function is abnormal then intracytoplasmic sperm injection (ICSI) is used in which a single sperm is selected and injected into each egg. For couples with normal sperm there is no advantage in using ICSI over IVF.

The inseminated eggs are left in the incubator overnight and checked for signs of fertilisation the next morning. On average, around 65 per cent of eggs fertilise normally and are then left in culture in the incubator. Sometimes, either no eggs are collected, or there are no mature eggs, or none fertilise normally, meaning that the cycle has sadly ended for the patient. More commonly, the fertilised eggs are cultured on. Incubators can be standard ones in which the embryologist takes the Petri dish out at intervals to check down a microscope for the development of each embryo, or time lapse, in which a camera is built within the incubator and takes an image at frequent intervals. The embryologist can assess development without needing to open the incubator door and move the embryos. In addition, certain developmental milestones that are associated with greater implantation potential, such as cells dividing within particular time frames, can be confirmed and used to aid embryo selection. The benefits of time-lapse systems in terms of increasing IVF success rates are yet to be fully established.

3. Blastocyst culture

Historically, most embryos were transferred at the cleavage stage (day 2 or 3) of development at which time they usually contain between 4 and 12 cells. With greater understanding of the nutritional and environmental requirements of embryos most centres now suggest culturing on to the blastocyst stage, day 5 to 6 of development, at which time they consist of 100–200 cells. Embryos that progress to be blastocysts have demonstrated greater implantation potential. It's not that the culturing itself has made the embryo 'better', it's that the embryo has shown itself to be so. Hence a random blastocyst will have a higher chance of success than a random cleavage stage (day 2 or 3) embryo. However, if a particular blastocyst had been identified on day 3 and transferred, the success rate would be the same. Hence, for patients who make only one or two embryos there would be little point in culturing to blastocyst since there is little choice in embryo selection. Blastocyst culture is a way of helping embryologists select between embryos, and to also transfer fewer embryos of higher potential. Therefore it is particularly useful for achieving high elective single embryo transfer (eSET) rates (with correspondingly low multiple birth rates) while maintaining an overall high pregnancy and live-birth rate.

4. Embryo transfer

The aim is to transfer one or two embryos via, the cervix, into the upper part of the uterine cavity. The woman is asked to have a full bladder, which has two benefits, though can be uncomfortable. The full bladder 1) pushes the main part of the uterus (the 'body') downwards, which straightens the angle between the canal of the cervix and uterus, and 2) acts as a 'window' onto the uterus for an abdominal ultrasound scan probe to be used during the ET procedure. Use of a scan in this way during ET has been shown to increase the IVF success rate. The embryologist, doctor or nurse will explain to the patient the embryo quality and a decision will be made on numbers of embryos to transfer. In the UK the HFEA allows a maximum of two embryos to be transferred in women under forty years of age and three for those women of forty years or more. While transferring greater numbers of embryos may increase the pregnancy rate slightly, it also significantly increases the risk of the most important complication of assisted conception, multiple birth. The HFEA has requested all IVF centres to change their practice to reduce to an overall multiple birth rate of less than 10 per cent per cycle. This is achieved by having an eSET policy such that patients at higher risk of multiple birth, for example younger age, first or second IVF cycle, and blastocyst transfer, only have a single embryo replaced. However, in the end the choice is usually down to the patient(s), though some NHS funding contracts may insist on eSET.

Following egg collection, it is necessary for the woman to take luteal support to aid implantation of the embryo(s). This is usually given by vaginal progesterone pessaries although the same hormone can be given rectally or by subcutaneous or intramuscular injection. The last option is not commonly used in the UK (much more so in the USA) as it isn't felt to be more successful but is associated with much more pain and a risk of severe infection (abscess). If pregnancy occurs, the luteal support can either be stopped on the day of the pregnancy test or continued until 7–12 weeks of pregnancy. Studies do not support continuing progesterone beyond the pregnancy test but the practice is widespread, probably for reassurance rather than anything else.

5. Embryo freezing

At the time of embryo transfer the 'best' one or two embryos are replaced. Very often there will be spare embryos of suitable quality that can be frozen for later use. The most successful technique is 'vitrification', in which embryos are 'snap-frozen' by plunging them into liquid nitrogen. Embryos can be stored at the cleavage (day 2–3) or blastocyst (day 5–6) stage. Blastocysts have greater implantation potential than cleavage stage embryos, hence many laboratories prefer to freeze only blastocysts. This reduces the numbers of embryos frozen so reducing costs for the patient and the subsequent frozen replacement success rate will be greater.

6. Frozen Embryo Replacement Cycles

A proportion of patients will have supernumerary embryos frozen from a fresh treatment or fertility preservation cycle (see below). When it comes to thawing and replacing the embryos the success (live-birth) rate is mainly dependent on the age of the woman at the time the embryos were frozen rather than her age (i.e. the age of her uterus) at the time of frozen transfer. It's as if her fertility has been 'frozen in time'. However, the frozen embryo(s) must be thawed and replaced into a receptive uterine environment. There are a number of different ways that this can be achieved. Women with regular ovulatory menstrual cycles have two main options: thawed embryos can be replaced in a natural menstrual cycle on the same cycle day that they would be arriving in the uterus during a natural conception; alternatively the uterus can be prepared with oestrogen tablets or patches to thicken the endometrium and then progesterone added to mimic the natural state after ovulation. After a few days of progesterone the embryo(s) are thawed and transferred. This latter approach may be called medicated, HRT, or programmed frozen cycles. If undertaking a medicated cycle it is important that the woman doesn't ovulate naturally as this would interfere with the hormone environment and timing of embryo replacement. Therefore, ovulation is either monitored for (and the cycle cancelled if it occurs), or a second drug used to prevent ovulation: the drugs used are either the GnRH agonist or antagonists (as used in the long and short fresh IVF protocols) respectively. If hormones are used to prepare the endometrium then it is necessary to continue the drugs into a pregnancy until the placenta has taken over. Most centres will continue to between 8 and 12 weeks gestation.

For women with regular ovulatory cycles the success rate with frozen replacement appears to be very similar between natural and medicated cycles. Therefore the choice may come down to the woman and her partner and how they feel about taking medication or not.

For women with irregular non-ovulatory cycles it is necessary to prepare the endometrium with drugs as described above.

7. Surgical Sperm Retrieval

Azoospermic (no sperm in the ejaculate) men may be offered a surgical sperm retrieval (SSR) in which sperm are taken directly from the testes or epididymis (tubes draining the testes) under anaesthetic. Sperm are then either frozen for later use in an IVF-ICSI cycle or used fresh. A problem with the latter approach is that both partners would need procedures performed on the same day, which could be logistically challenging, and also there would be the risk that no sperm is retrieved, giving the couple little time to consider options such as donor insemination. As there is no negative effect on IVF-ICSI success rates of using frozen compared to fresh testicular sperm many clinics prefer the first approach. There are a number of different techniques used. Very often the first and simplest approach is to use either a needle or 'tru-cut' biopsy instrument directly into the testis to remove a number of tubules. These are then examined down the microscope by the scientist for sperm within. Sperm can also be extracted from the epididymis (PESA: Percutaneous Epididymal Sperm Aspiration). Some believe that epididymal sperm, being more mature than sperm retrieved from the testis, should be used in preference though studies do not support that view.

The SSR can also be performed as an open procedure by making a full incision through the layers of the scrotum and removing small pieces of testicular tissue. The total volume of tissue removed is generally greater with an open compared to needle approach and may be preferred for men who have a degree of testicular failure (noted by raised levels of FSH, low levels of testosterone, and small testes). A more recent development is micro-TESA in which, during an open operation, a testis is opened (almost divided) and a high-power operating microscope used by the surgeon to try and identify pockets of sperm production within the testicular tissue. Risks of SSR include pain, bruising, bleeding and permanent testicular damage including a very low risk of subsequent testicular failure.

The likelihood of finding sperm with an SSR mostly depends on the degree of testicular failure. Men who have normal functioning testes (normal FSH and testosterone levels, and normal testicular sizes on examination) should have sperm retrieval rates of 80–100 per cent. For men with testicular failure the pickup rate depends on the degree of failure and decreases with increasing FSH levels and decreasing testicular volume.

8. Preimplantation Genetic Screening (PGS) and Diagnosis (PGD)

A normal human embryo has 23 pairs of chromosomes. However, on average, around half of embryos that couples make, whether naturally or during IVF, will contain the wrong numbers of chromosomes. The abnormality usually arises in the egg or sperm and is then passed on into the embryo. The proportion of abnormal embryos produced increases with a woman's age. Such embryos usually don't implant (hence it takes, on average, longer for a woman to conceive as she ages) but, if they do implant, most will miscarry in the first trimester (first twelve weeks of pregnancy). The combination of a lower chance of implantation (i.e. lower chance of a positive pregnancy test) and a higher chance of miscarriage, results in a significant decline in the chance of live birth per cycle of either trying naturally or per fertility treatment cycle.

While most pregnancies affected by incorrect numbers of chromosomes do not continue beyond the first trimester, some do. Down syndrome (three chromosome number 21s) is one example and so much of the screening offered to women between 12 and 16 weeks is to diagnose Down syndrome and then to consider options of continuing with the pregnancy or termination.

One option is to examine the genetic status of the embryo(s) before transfer back to the uterus. During a PGS cycle the couple undergo standard IVF treatment and embryos are cultured to the blastocyst stage. With a laser or chemicals, a hole is made in the outer shell of the blastocyst and three to five cells removed from the trophectoderm (the part of the blastocyst that goes on to develop into the placenta). The cells are then either analysed over the next 24 hours using a technique called array-CGH which allows for a fresh transfer on day 6, or the biopsied embryos are vitrified (frozen) while the cells are analysed by Next Generation Sequencing (NGS) which takes longer. Chromosomally normal embryos can then be transferred in a subsequent frozen embryo replacement cycle.

The benefits of PGS are currently unclear. If a couple produce, for example, five blastocysts which are all frozen and replaced one-by-one then, at some point, a chromosomally normal embryo, if present, will be replaced. If, instead, PGS was used before the embryos were frozen, then any chromosomally normal embryos would be replaced earlier without going through unnecessary FER cycles with abnormal embryos being transferred. Hence, the chance of live birth per egg collection is likely to be the same with or without PGS, but PGS may shorten the time to success (identification and replacement of any normal embryos produced) and reduce the number of failed FER cycles and miscarriages. The results of larger studies are awaited.

A similar technique to PGS is Preimplantation Genetic Diagnosis (PGD). The approach taken during an IVF cycle is the same as detailed above, but PGD is used in families who have an inherited genetic condition rather than just screening embryos from otherwise healthy parents as is the case with PGS. The cells taken from the blastocyst are analysed for the single gene defect, for example cystic fibrosis. In the UK the HFEA list the genetic conditions for which clinics can perform PGD. For a new condition the clinic applies to the HFEA and a multi-team review, including ethicists, scientists and the public, comment before a decision is made on whether the condition should be added to the permitted list.

9. Additional Techniques

9.1 Endometrial scratch

Some studies suggest that embryo implantation rate is increased by causing a minor degree of temporary trauma to the endometrial lining in the cycle before treatment. A thin plastic catheter, most commonly a 'Pipelle', is passed through the cervix via a speculum and moved to the top of the endometrial cavity. The inner part of the Pipelle is then pulled-back to create a vacuum and some endometrial cells are sucked into the outer Pipelle. The whole catheter is then withdrawn. Originally the Pipelle was designed to biopsy the endometrium of, for example, post-menopausal women with unusual bleeding for cancer. Small IVF studies suggest that the procedure can improve the implantation rate, though numbers of patients in the studies are limited and more data are required on the true effect and, importantly, who would benefit the most, for example, women with a number of failed cycles.

9.2 Embryo glue

Small studies suggest that embryos that are bathed in a particular composition of culture media, containing high concentrations of hyaluronan, on the morning of embryo transfer have a greater implantation rate. Larger studies are required to confirm the initial findings.

9.3 Time lapse incubators

During routine IVF embryologists remove embryos from their incubator every other day or so to examine development and quality using a microscope. The change in temperature and surroundings can be potentially detrimental. Also, the analyses are only 'snap shots' during the days of development in the laboratory. An alternative method is to leave the embryos in the incubator and to take digital images every few minutes with an inbuilt camera. The resulting video is then analysed automatically by computer to assess which embryos reach developmental stages (for example 8 cells) at optimal time points and also allowing the embryologists to assess quality while the embryos remain in the incubator. Some studies suggest that use of time lapse incubators improves outcome but, as with many new developments in IVF (including those described above), the studies tend to be too small ('underpowered') and to have methodological flaws which mean that results need to be treated with caution.

10. Conclusion

The success rates of IVF have been slowly but surely increasing over the last forty years. In addition, the treatment is safer than before due to the push to reduce the rates of multiple birth (by improving embryo culture and selection techniques so that eSET can be used) and OHSS (by using short antagonist cycles plus agonist triggers in high risk women). There are a number of fairly recent developments available for patients to 'bolt-on' to the main IVF cycle, usually for an extra cost, and rarely funded by the NHS (as described above). However, there is a dearth of good-quality studies examining many of the newer additional techniques, which hampers decision making for couples and clinicians. A number of large, properly conducted studies are beginning to examine these areas so, within the next few years, the situation should become clearer.

IVF is an established and successful treatment for infertility. Hopefully this chapter, by explaining the process of an IVF cycle and the various additional techniques available, will aid in decision making for those considering moving on to treatment.

CHAPTER 3

PREPARE YOUR MIND TO PREPARE YOUR BODY

Alison Leverett-Morris BA (Hons), MA, ADHP,
NSHP&M, UKCP
Integrative hypno-psychotherapist, specialising in
fertility and mind-body health and wellbeing

1. Introduction

When I heard the words 'Congratulations, that's wonderful'
I was bewildered. Congratulations were not in order and
it most definitely was not wonderful. I'd just told a work
colleague I was about to start IVF. As I look back on that
moment, more than eighteen years later, I understand
why I found it upsetting. I hadn't come to terms with
the disappointment and losses I'd undergone and I felt
that my painful experiences were being dismissed. And
yet, I too was treating the pain of infertility as something
best ignored.

Some six years after that 'incident' I remember telling

a good friend that I was about to start IVF (again). She also said, 'That's wonderful', but this time I was in full agreement. It was wonderful. So what had changed? In short, I had. My husband had. 'We' had. We were ready, we were hopeful and we were grateful. Grateful for the personal growth we experienced as a result of our fertility journey and grateful to live in a time when modern medicine gave us the chance of the family we hoped for. That was wonderful. For everyone about to embark on IVF, that is wonderful. A healthy mindset can transform the way you experience IVF.

As a hypnotherapist and psychotherapist, my personal path to becoming a parent brings empathy and integrity to my professional practice. I understand the emotional investment IVF involves and genuinely seek to utilise the most ethical, effective and evidence-based therapeutic interventions. My focus is on solutions and outcomes for the individuals and couples that I work with.

I invite you to embrace a solution-focused approach to *your* IVF cycle. It is my privilege to offer information, insights and tools that may help you to set yourself up for IVF success. Some of the suggestions may inspire, guide and support you. Others may not. As the saying goes: 'one man's treasure is another man's trash'. Notice what resonates for *you*. Notice what makes you stop and think about something a little differently. Trust what feels right for you. Find treasure.

2. Acknowledge what hurts

It may seem paradoxical to talk about what hurts in the context of a solution-focused approach to fertility and IVF. But acknowledging the emotional pain you feel is an important first step. Prepare your mind to prepare your body. Of course, when pain is ignored it can sometimes go away or get better on its own. But, just like toothache, it can also flare up when you least want it.

The impact of fertility problems is often underestimated and misunderstood. For most people, IVF is not the first port of call to having a family. IVF is often experienced after long months or years of trying to conceive naturally, undergoing medical investigations and trying less invasive fertility treatments. This may be at significant emotional, physical and financial cost. Powerful and unresolved emotions resulting from the grief, losses and disappointments of fertility problems and/or miscarriage may be present. And so starting IVF does not feel the same as starting to try for a baby. IVF isn't the beginning. There is often a lot of painful 'water under the bridge' by that point. It may still hurt.

In my clinical practice, many of the individuals and couples that I work with feel the painful aspects of their fertility problems are 'glossed over' by the people in their lives. It is equally common for people to gloss over their own pain. There can be a lot of 'cheering up', 'looking on the bright side' and 'other people have it far worse' going on. Sometimes those who squash down unwanted emotions, with a determination to think positively, find they experience an increase in unhealthy coping mechanisms (such as comfort eating, smoking or drinking). Others find they are unexpectedly 'floored' by an experience such as a friend's pregnancy announcement.

If any of this resonates with you it's likely that emotional pain is present and needs to be acknowledged. When you acknowledge what hurts, your perspective will change and you can begin to positively transform the way you experience IVF. What follows are my top three tips for how to do this:

2.1 Tip 1: Accept that people respond differently to experiencing or witnessing emotional pain

Recall a time when you saw or heard someone cry out in pain after an accident or injury... maybe someone slicing a finger while chopping vegetables or a child falling off a swing. What was your initial response? Did anyone else present respond in the same way or did they respond differently?

Some people find it very difficult when they see that somebody has been physically injured. They will literally hide their eyes or block their ears to avoid being confronted with the source of the other person's pain. The fear of what it might 'be like' can be overwhelming. And yet others will go straight to the source of the pain, take a good look and do whatever needs doing to make it better.

Likewise, we don't all respond in the same way to our own physical pain. Some of us ignore pain and hope it will go away. Some of us cannot bear to look at the source of our pain, but are willing to seek help and allow a doctor or somebody else to look at it. Some of us take a close look to see if it's something we can fix ourselves or whether help is required.

The same is true of psychological or emotional pain. It's a fact that some people find it very difficult to look at, or even hear about, what hurts – regardless of whether the pain is their own or someone else's. Accepting this fact can change your whole outlook and experience of IVF. It enables you to begin to let go of feeling hurt, disappointed or angry at the way your mum, best friend or partner is responding to your emotional distress. It enables you to forgive *your* response to emotional pain.

2.2 Tip 2: Ditch the painkillers – pain is your ally

Pain is often treated as an unwelcome guest – we want to get away from it or have that 'guest' leave as soon as possible. Such attitudes can make it difficult to examine or soothe the pain – and may even perpetuate the symptoms. Pain is a useful warning signal. Pain directs attention towards the location and nature of the situation, thought or behaviour that needs to be changed. Pain shines a spotlight on whatever is preventing or interfering with our comfort and motivates us to seek help. In this way, pain is our ally.

Viewing pain as your ally can transform your experience of IVF. Pain is not something to be 'killed'; it is something to be listened to and utilised. When you listen to pain's whisper it no longer needs to shout.

2.3 Tip 3: Allow the source of your pain to point to its solution

When it comes to pain and determining how to move towards a more comfortable position, there is nobody better positioned or qualified than you are. In my clinical practice I often begin treatment by facilitating a 'diagnostic trance' to create change quickly and efficiently. This is something you can do yourself, by following these steps:

1. Become aware of an emotional 'pain', relating to IVF, that you would prefer not to have. For example, feeling that the fertility problems are 'all your fault'.

2. Close your eyes and take slow comfortable breaths. Allow yourself to begin to relax.

3. Begin to concentrate on the unpleasant feelings or sensations that you associate with the problem you have identified. (Just as, when we lie in bed at night, our attention can be drawn to physical aches and pains that we didn't notice during our busy day.)

4. Observe and pay very close attention to what you feel, without trying to think of anything else at all.

5. Continue to focus on those unpleasant feelings and observe whatever thoughts, words or images pop into your head. (It may be that a seemingly unrelated image or a previously forgotten incident will spring to mind.) If you feel stuck, simply focus on physical feelings. Do you feel tightness in your throat or a weight in your chest? Focusing on such feelings may lead you to associations and further thoughts.

6. Find a pleasant thought or image that moves or removes the unpleasant feelings, images, words, memory or thoughts that arose in association with the unpleasant feelings. Allow your unconscious to communicate this to you as a solution. (If you are finding this difficult, simply imagine how it might feel if the unpleasant feeling were gone.)

Many of us will be surprised to discover that at an unconscious level we know exactly what we can do to resolve an emotional problem we are experiencing. Very often this procedure will reveal the internal events responsible for the discomfort and lead to a decision to change a self-limiting habit, an outdated belief or unhelpful behaviour.

3. Manage expectations

It isn't easy to manage your expectations of IVF when there is so much conflicting advice about what to expect:

Expect it to work first time. Don't expect it to work first time. Expect IVF to bring you closer to your partner. Expect IVF to wreck your relationship. Many people find it helpful to be told to expect the IVF route to parenthood to be a challenge. Others find this disconcerting.

Expectations can lurk in our subconscious without us even knowing they are there. When we find somebody's advice on what to expect helpful, it is usually because it matches what we are already expecting at a subconscious level (or it is compatible with our general world view or outlook on life). When we find somebody's advice hard to swallow, it is usually because it conflicts with our subconscious expectations (or it's incompatible with our general world view or outlook on life).

Top tip: Be alert to mismatches

Have you ever picked up a dish only to drop it straight back down because it was burning hot and it hurt? You expected the dish to be cool but it wasn't.

This is an example of a mismatch between your expectation and your experience – and the mismatch hurt. Pain is like an alarm going off. Pain alerts you when your expectation differs from your experience. The same can be true of emotional pain. Sometimes the cause of the emotional pain you experience on your fertility journey is a mismatch between your expectation and your experience.

I've picked up a hot dish many times, most of us have! Usually our pain response is fast enough for us to drop the dish before we get seriously burnt. When the 'pain alarm' sounds, we can stop the pain by aligning our expectation and experience. We do this by making a choice: change our expectation or change the experience. In this example, both options are available to us: we can expect the dish to be hot (and so wear an oven glove) or we can change the experience (wait for the dish to cool down). In life, it isn't always possible to change the experience. With IVF, many experiences are outside our control. When this is the case, the solution is to change your expectation.

Here is a simple technique that can help you to change unhelpful or unrealistic expectations that are causing you pain.

1. When the 'pain alarm' sounds, become aware of what is causing you pain.

    For example: I feel upset because Julie keeps rubbing it in about how wonderful it is to be pregnant.

2. Become aware of what you are saying to yourself (your inner dialogue).

For example: I'm so angry with her, she obviously doesn't care about my feelings.

3. Rate your level of disturbance when you think this thought (where 10 is the worst it could be and 0 is no disturbance at all).

For example: This is definitely an 8, she's my sister, I can't believe she is so insensitive.

4. Ask yourself: 'What are your expectations about this situation?' (Note, this stage might take some time: our expectations aren't always obvious and often it's necessary to move through many layers of expectation before you find the 'hidden' one that is causing the pain.)

For example: I'm expecting Julie to be more sensitive about my feelings... (after deeper thought)... As the older sister I have always expected to be the first to have a baby.

5. Rate your level of disturbance with this expectation.

For example: This is still an 8. It's really painful, I feel like my younger sister's life is moving on and mine isn't.

6. Ask yourself: Is the solution to change your expectation or change the experience?

For example: I can't change the experience — my sister is already pregnant before me — I can only change my expectation.

7. How would your expectation need to change in order to bring that level of disturbance down?

For example: I can accept that life doesn't always go to plan and expect my life to follow its own unique path.

8. How does that expectation change your level of disturbance when you think about your sister being pregnant?

For example: It's a 3. I'm no longer expecting to be able to control the order of life events.

4. Create a healthy mindset

A healthy mindset can enhance your fertility and dramatically reduce any negative impacts of IVF. There is a plethora of scientific evidence showing a relationship between psychological factors and physical health. Our minds and bodies are in constant communication – they are not separate entities. Our bodies respond to what is happening in our minds and our minds respond to what is happening in our bodies. A mind-body approach to fertility, such as hypnotherapy, is one that *purposely* uses the mind to influence positive changes in the body – and vice versa.

Molecules in the body (called neuropeptides) inform the body on how to respond to thoughts and feelings. Quite literally, these 'molecule messengers' communicate thoughts into physical responses.

Experience your neuropeptides at work

Imagine that you are holding a fresh, ripe lemon. In your imagination, concentrate intently on that lemon – notice what it feels like, looks like and smells like. Begin to imagine that in a few moments' time you'll rest the lemon on a chopping board, take a knife and slowly cut the lemon into small pieces. As you do so, the citrus smell fills the room and you feel the sticky juice on your fingers. You are now slowly lifting a piece of lemon towards your mouth. You notice the fresh citrus smell as you slowly bring the juicy, dripping segment of lemon closer and closer to your mouth. And as you experience the sharp, acidic taste, you notice that your mouth is watering more and more...

Most people who take 'the lemon test' will salivate – and this is an excellent example of how thoughts alone can trigger a physical response.

Of course, we are not consciously aware of all our physiological responses because many are very subtle. Furthermore, science has not yet advanced to the extent that we can identify every subtle physiological response in our bodies. But just because we are not aware of something, that doesn't mean it isn't happening. There is robust scientific evidence that the body responds according to how we are thinking and feeling. So, in relation to IVF, how you are thinking and feeling is very important.

Some women tell themselves that their IVF cycle will fail in the hope of avoiding disappointment if it does. This is a faulty strategy. Firstly, disappointment is still felt when an IVF cycle fails. Secondly, you are sending a negative message to your body. Do you really want your neuropeptides to be telling your body to respond to the message: 'I'm not going to get pregnant'? ... Imagine how differently your body may respond to messages such as 'My body is healthy, equipped and ready to nurture and receive our embryo'.

- Soroka Medical Centre in Israel found using hypnosis during embryo transfer achieved 53 per cent clinical pregnancies compared to 32 per cent in regular IVF cycles.

- Harvard Medical Centre, USA, found that visualisation and mind-body techniques increased pregnancy rates and outcome in both natural and assisted conception.

If you are interested in using mind-body techniques to enhance the key stages of your IVF cycle, I encourage you to seek out a suitably qualified practitioner to work with face-to-face or through online resources. The clinical application of hypnosis can literally change the way you think by encouraging the creation of new neural pathways.

In changing how you think, you can change how your mind and body communicate with each other. There is so much you can do to create a healthy mindset for IVF treatment. I am delighted to share with you three ideas that I have seen can make a difference.

4.1 Tip 1: Body and mind

Your intention is a powerful thing. It's the psychological equivalent of typing the postcode of your desired destination into a satnav. Your intention is the message you send to your mind and your body. When you are undergoing IVF, your body receives medication to trigger physiological responses that enable and support a pregnancy. When you intend to become pregnant you allow mind and body to align, giving you the very best chance of success. Be clear on what IVF success means for *you*.

Let's imagine that Rachel has just booked a flight to Sydney, Australia. For as long as she can remember, Rachel has dreamed of doing a bungee jump off Sydney Harbour Bridge. She's been saving up for years and can't wait to get there and do the jump!

Let's imagine Sarah has just booked a flight to Sydney, Australia. The Australian lifestyle has always appealed to Sarah and she's really looking forward to experiencing it. Sydney is her preferred destination because she has dreamed of doing a bungee jump off of Sydney Harbour Bridge for as long as she can remember. However, Sarah intends to get as much out of this trip as possible. She intends to fly from London to Amsterdam to spend a few days with an old friend. She has ideas of places she'd like to visit in Amsterdam, but her main intention is to have fun with her friend. Sarah intends to fly from Amsterdam to Sydney, but will stop over in Singapore. Sarah hopes to learn as much about Singaporean culture as possible before catching her connecting flight to Sydney. Sarah has thoroughly researched places of interest in Sydney and the bungee jump is still top of her list of intentions – but she has no fixed itinerary. Sarah intends to experience as much as possible while in Sydney.

Let's now imagine that Sydney Harbour Bridge is closed for maintenance. It's inevitable that both Rachel and Sarah will be very disappointed. However, it is most likely that only Rachel will feel she's made an unsuccessful trip.

When you are thinking about what IVF success means to you – be Sarah.

It's not for me, or anyone else for that matter, to tell you what IVF success means for you. But of course, a baby is most people's idea of a successful IVF cycle. Hold on to your desire for a baby and see this as your hope and your intention. But don't 'be Rachel'. Have many positive intentions for your IVF cycle.

In my experience, clear, positive and purposeful intentions are the foundation of a healthy mindset for IVF success. I have seen benefit from the following: taking some time to build a clear mental picture of what IVF success looks like for the person undergoing the treatment. Intending to maintain a close loving relationship with their partner. Intending to enjoy time with friends. Intending to eat well, sleep well and live well. When they are clear on their intentions they are purposely intending to succeed.

4.2 Tip 2: Goals that align with intentions

We have a basic human need to progress and move forward in life, while also feeling competent and able to manage the situations we find ourselves in. When goals are realistic and achievable, we are motivated to continue moving forwards. When something is too far out of our comfort zone or simply cannot be achieved through effort or persistence, the effect is frustration and loss of confidence in our abilities to succeed.

Resilience gives us the ability to thrive, mature and continue to move forward with confidence whatever the prevailing circumstances. Resilience is therefore a very important attribute for IVF success. Achieving goals helps to build resilience. And this is why setting healthy goals is such an important part of creating a healthy mindset for IVF success.

When setting goals for IVF success it is important to separate out your intentions from your goals. A healthy goal is something that we have control over. We don't always have control over our intentions. This is why pregnancy is a great intention, but it is not a healthy goal, because unfortunately pregnancy cannot be guaranteed, and nor can we control the outcome of pregnancy.

A metaphor for understanding the difference between an intention and a goal

Let's just imagine for a moment that you have been living in a high-rise flat. You've been happy living here and generally just 'getting on with your life', but in the back of your mind you've always had a desire to grow vegetables in your own garden. When the circumstances in your life change, and you have a garden of your own, you decide that now, you want to grow your own vegetables more than ever. So, let's think of that as your intention. It cannot be your goal because none of us has control over the actual growth of the vegetables. However, there is a lot we can do to encourage the growth of these vegetables.

The *intention* is to grow vegetables. The *goal* is to create an environment that gives the vegetables the very best chance of growing. Goals might include: buying the best-quality seeds from a reputable buyer, finding out about the optimal pH balance of soil, preparing the soil accordingly, planting the seeds at the appropriate time of year, finding out how to best support the growth of the seeds and feeding and watering accordingly. All of these goals are achievable and in alignment with the intention. By achieving these goals we increase the likelihood of the vegetables flourishing. But at the same time, we understand that we cannot control the actual growth of the vegetables.

When setting goals for IVF success, begin by being clear on your intentions (that which you hope for, but cannot guarantee or control). Then, set achievable goals that support and align with your intentions.

4.3 Tip 3: Being clear on goals

If we are to stay motivated and achieve our goals, we need to know what it is that we're aiming for. Asking ourselves what will be different when the goals have been achieved? How will we know that we have achieved the goal? What will others notice about us when we have achieved our goal? This solution-focused thinking helps us to build a clear picture of how we will be thinking, feeling and behaving in our goal state. I have seen these four simple ideas help with this process:

1. Identify the change that needs to be made (for example: *'I need to change the way that I withdraw from my friends during IVF because this makes me feel isolated and lonely'*).

2. Orientating goals towards the outcome and the change that we want (solution focused rather than problem focused. For example: *'I want to feel connected to my friends and interested in what's going on in the world beyond my IVF cycle'*).

3. Ensuring that goals are good at drawing out our strengths and resources (for example: *'I have good organisation skills, I have enough money for at least one night out a month'*).

4. Visualising what it is like when we have achieved our goal (for example: *'I am going for a walk with my friend Suzy one lunchtime a week, I am going out for dinner with friends once a month, I am joining in with the conversations on my WhatsApp messages'*.

When you have a clear visual image of your goal state you can then identify the 'steps along the way' that will get you there. These steps are your goals. To continue with the above example, one goal could be *'By the end of the day I will message Suzy asking if she'd like to go for a walk with me, once a week, during our lunch hour'*. This is a healthy goal that is aligned with the intention of feeling connected to friends.

Healthy goals are always SMART – which means they are Specific, they can be Measured and they are Achievable, Realistic, and Time specific. Look again at the above example of a healthy goal: this goal is specific (I will message Suzy), it is measurable (you either send the message or you don't), it is achievable, realistic and time specific (by the end of the day). It is a goal aligned with the intention to feel connected with friends.

For IVF success, goals should always align with your 'big picture' intention. Writing goals down and displaying them somewhere where we will see them often. Clear, realistic and achievable goals are the building blocks of a healthy mindset for IVF success. Feel your motivation, optimism and confidence soar as you work towards – and achieve – your goals.

5. Maintain a healthy mindset

Having created a healthy mindset for IVF success, you will undoubtedly want to keep it. The good news is that you can train your brain to maintain a healthy mindset effortlessly and automatically. Focusing on your goals every day will help you to achieve this.

A daily practice of focusing on your goals will, quite literally, change how you experience IVF. You will find yourself noticing all the good things in your life, you will find yourself becoming aware of all that you are doing to support your fertility and you will find yourself noticing evidence of your fertility health more and more. The more you notice these things the more motivated and resilient you become. And the more motivated and resilient you become, the more able you are to achieve your goals whatever the 'weather'. You are in an excellent mindset for IVF success.

I understand that it takes effort to focus on your goals daily – and that it's easy for practices such as this to fall off the agenda when life gets busy. To commit to something, we have to believe it's going to be worth the effort. We need to understand the 'why'? If we don't understand *why* something is important or helpful, we're not likely to commit to it. So here's the science bit...

We all have something called a Reticular Activating System (RAS). This is a bundle of nerves at the back of our head, the central core of the brain stem. The RAS has the ability to filter out information and so it plays a big role in what we see, hear and notice every day.

We have all experienced the RAS at work

I'm not interested in cars. I like driving and I like going places, but I'm not one of those people that enjoy owning (or aspiring to own) a certain make or model of car. To me, they're just cars and pretty much all look the same. I don't generally take much notice of them.

A few days ago I was flicking through the newsfeed on my phone and I happened to read that car sales had fallen slightly last year and the highest-selling car in the UK was the Ford Fiesta. Later that day I was going about my normal business and Ford Fiestas were everywhere. I'd stop at a red light and the car in front would be a Ford Fiesta. I'd park my car and there'd be a Ford Fiesta right next to me. I went to visit a friend and, you guessed it, that 'red car' I've seen a thousand times on her driveway was a Ford Fiesta. They were everywhere!

This was my RAS at work. My RAS ensured that I noticed those Ford Fiestas because it 'thought' it was important to me.

The RAS works like this: every moment of every day we are bombarded with information. The subconscious mind can process up to 40 million bits of data per second. The conscious mind only has the capacity to process up to 40 bits of data per second. In order to function well, we need those 40 things in our conscious mind to be relevant and important to the particular circumstances of every given moment. We need a system to filter out the most important information.

The RAS is that system, for it acts like a gatekeeper to the conscious mind. The RAS only lets through information that is of interest to the conscious mind. When something is dominant in our conscious thoughts, the RAS 'thinks', *'This must be important, so I'll "open the gate" and let everything related to that important thought through. Everything else can stay on the other side of the gate'* (out of awareness in the subconscious). This is why, for example, if you frequently think thoughts such as *'I'm the only one that can't get pregnant'*, it will seem as if everybody is pregnant apart from you – you will notice pregnant women everywhere. Your RAS is trying to help you, it thinks 'seeing pregnancy everywhere' is important to you.

One last idea for maintaining a healthy mindset for IVF success

Always focus on your intentions and your goals with emotion. If you strongly desire to have a baby, and that is your intention, FEEL that desire when you *purposely* intend to succeed. And when you are focusing on your goals, FEEL the emotion of what will be different when you have achieved the goal. Your RAS doesn't listen to half-hearted instructions. Your RAS always listens to heart-felt instructions.

This is why it is so important to be clear on what you want (your intention) and to focus on it daily (your goals). In doing this, you are deliberately programming your RAS. You are quite literally telling your RAS, as gatekeeper of those 40 billion bits of data, what you want to let through to your conscious mind. And this is why you recognise those things, people, resources, examples and ideas that will help you achieve your goal.

Quite simply, when you programme your RAS to work for you, life is better. This is the sort of shift I witness so often in my clinical practice:

(Start of therapy): Julie frequently says things like... *'It's so obvious I'm going to be one of those people that stays "unexplained" and never gets pregnant'* ... *'the success rates for IVF are so low it's not really worth me bothering'* ... *'everywhere I go people are pregnant, and they are all younger than me'* ... *'I just don't feel fertile'*...

(After purposely intending to succeed and focusing daily on her goals): Julie comes to sessions saying things like... *'I felt a sensation the other day and wondered if I was ovulating and sure enough when I took a test, I was'* ... *'I feel so much more energetic these days, I reckon I'm healthier now than I was five years ago'* ... *'I heard about this woman the other day that got pregnant on her first IVF cycle and she was older than me'*...

6. Manage stress

Entering 'how to manage stress' into a search engine will return around 300 million results. Stress management techniques can be very effective and are not difficult to find. I believe it is also useful to consider the way that you *view* stress. I share an example from my clinical practice that I hope will prompt you to think differently about your capabilities and capacity to manage stress during your IVF cycle.

Isabel came to me some months prior to starting her first IVF cycle. She is a fit and healthy individual, with a career she enjoys, a happy relationship and good friends. We worked through her fears and anxieties, related to years of trying unsuccessfully to conceive, and Isabel was in a very healthy mindset before starting IVF.

Isabel knew that the week before starting her IVF medication she would be flying to South Asia to speak at a conference and lead a five-day training course. She was looking forward to this trip and was resourced with mind-body techniques that would support her to manage the particulars of her circumstances.

A few days before the flight, Isabel was advised by a professional (working in the fertility field) not to make the trip because the psychological and physical stressors involved would impair her chance of IVF success. I'm not in the habit of criticising other professionals or different approaches to enhancing fertility. However, in the interests of reassuring anyone reading this (who may need to travel during IVF), I feel it important to note that this advice did *not* come from Isabel's doctor or anyone at the fertility clinic that was treating her.

Isabel 'swallowed this advice whole' and lost sight of her coping capacity. She spiralled into a highly stressed state and was on the brink of cancelling her trip. This would have significant consequences for her career and her relationship, which of course would lead to further stress (Isabel and her partner worked for the same company and had agreed not to tell their employer they were having IVF).

For many people, a long-haul flight, speaking at a conference and running a training course would be the epitome of stress. But for Isabel these things nourish her soul. A long-haul flight is when Isabel catches up on sleep! By simply reminding Isabel of her personal strengths and preferences, she was able to apply a healthy filter to the advice she had been given and remember how brilliantly resourced she was to cope.

Isabel made the trip – and some months later she had a beautiful baby girl.

6.1 Filter other people's advice (and that includes mine!)

It's great to be well informed on what can give you the best chance of IVF success. But have you ever heard the saying *one man's cure is another man's poison*? When it comes to advice – that's my advice. Not all 'good advice' is good for *you*. Following every piece of advice in an attempt to have 'the perfect IVF' can be a great cause of stress.

Stress is an imbalance between the demands of the environment and the person's coping capacity. This varies from person to person. Not everything that appears stressful *is* stressful. It is only stressful if it's beyond your ability to cope. You can save yourself a whole heap of stress by applying a 'healthy filter' to advice that you are given. Know yourself. Know your coping capacity. Many 'stressful' things are well within your coping capacity.

6.2 Don't stress about stress

Science shows there is a relationship between psychological stress and fertility. Advances in scientific understanding enable the mind-body relationship to be better understood. And as a result, mind-body approaches to fertility such as hypnotherapy are increasingly popular. Mind-body techniques are at the very core of my professional practice and so it may seem strange for me to say to you: don't stress about stress.

Fertility problems are rarely, if ever, caused by one single factor. You may or may not have an identified 'reason' for being referred for IVF; perhaps it is low sperm count, a blocked tube or something else. Even when a 'reason' is identified, this is not the full picture of your fertility health. There are many factors that contribute to fertility health. Some of these factors are within our control (for example, whether or not we smoke). Other factors we cannot control (for example, our age or genes). And, of course, the full picture of fertility health includes *all* contributory factors of *both* partners (and donors too, when having IVF with donor gametes).

And so while there is evidence of how psychological stress affects fertility, it is important to remember that stress is *one* factor in a bigger picture. Every day, babies are conceived and born in acutely and chronically stressful circumstances, such as rape, famine and war. This levelling thought can help to maintain perspective on the relationship between stress and fertility.

Mostly, I work with people in preparation for, and during, IVF. But from time to time someone will make first contact in the late stages of their IVF cycle. This is often because they want help to 'undo the damage' of a stressful event such as a row with their partner. It saddens me to see the enormous pressure these individuals have put themselves under to have the 'perfect stress-free IVF'. And sadly, the effort of trying not to get stressed is often the biggest cause of their stress.

Life is unpredictable and there is so much we cannot control. Stuff happens. As and when a challenge crops up, I urge you – please don't stress about the stress. At risk of repeating myself, I'll say it again: fertility problems are rarely, if ever, caused by one single factor. Every day, babies are conceived and born in acutely and chronically stressful circumstances.

6.3 Prioritise excellent self-care

Self-care is vitally important if you are to achieve and maintain optimal mind-body health before, during and after IVF. We are most prone to stress overload when we have a lack of control over our circumstances and lack the vital skills or resources to cope with those circumstances. There is much we cannot control about IVF. But we *can* develop the skills and resources to cope. And we *can* plan in advance how we can best support ourselves.

Self-care builds resilience by ensuring you have emotional reserves to draw on. I like to think of this in terms of a wellbeing bank account. Positive experiences and relaxation put 'funds' into the bank account. Negative, tiring or difficult experiences take 'funds' out of the bank account. Excellent self-care means that you budget carefully and wherever possible you 'live within your means'.

Some of us habitually practise good self-care. Some of us don't. Some of us feel we need to earn a 'treat' like a massage or a leisurely soak in the bath. Some of us view these things as a life essential. If you are someone that tends to 'soldier on' without reward I encourage you to make self-care your top priority during IVF.

Here is how to keep a wellbeing bank account:

Step 1. Create your bank account in a notebook or a spreadsheet, whatever works best for you. But ALWAYS keep a written log. Trust me, mental calculations just don't work because they can't highlight patterns of behaviour over time or show the cumulative balance of wellbeing.

Step 2. Take a moment to sit quietly, close your eyes, take a few slow breaths and make an honest assessment of your current state of stress. Give this a score between 0 and 10 (10 being highly stressed). Let's say your score is 7. So, £7 is your 'opening balance', the amount of 'money' you have in your wellbeing bank account.

Step 3. At the end of every day, log 'income' and 'expenditure'. Positive experiences and relaxation are income. Negative or tiring experiences are expenditure. The 'price' depends on the intensity of the experience. You might score something that was really good fun as £5 income. Something difficult, but not too bad, you might score as £2 expenditure. For ease keep the prices of 'normal day-to-day life' within a £10 limit. But of course, if something very significant happens, like a miscarriage or winning the lottery, you may feel this merits a far higher amount.

Your log can be as brief or as detailed as you like. Below is an example of what it could look like.

Step 4. Most events, as shown below, will 'sit' within a single day. But if you are affected by an event over a number of days, weeks or months, then be sure to log the 'price' on a daily basis. For example, if (as per the example below) you continue to be upset by your colleague's pregnancy, then for every day that it negatively affects you, log it as negative expenditure – in addition to what else happens each day.

Step 5. When keeping your log, beware of 'shoulds' or 'shouldn'ts'. Notice if you find yourself saying things like 'I should be happy for my colleague', 'I shouldn't log her pregnancy as a negative experience'. Forget shoulds and shouldn'ts. The purpose of this exercise is to log how you *actually* feel – not how you believe you 'should' feel.

Step 6. You may find your wellbeing bank account highlights that certain situations are affecting you on a daily basis over a long period. This awareness may prompt you to make decisions about how you might resolve the negative emotions surrounding that situation, for example by seeing a professional therapist.

Step 7. Always carry over the end-of-week balance into the following week. This is now your opening balance for that week.

An example of a wellbeing 'bank account':

Opening balance: £7

Income

Monday	£1 (nice chat and cuddle with John)
Tuesday	£2 (walk at lunchtime, after-work swim)
Wednesday	£1 (John cooked dinner)
Thursday	£2 (nice bath and early night with my book)
Friday	£1 (walk at lunchtime)
Saturday	£5 (day at spa with best friend)
Sunday	£3 (cycle ride and pub lunch with John)
Total	£15

Expenditure

Monday	£2 (tough day at work)
Tuesday	£5 (work colleague announces pregnancy on first month of trying to conceive)
Wednesday	£0 (nothing negative today)
Thursday	£2 (invited to friend's baby shower, not in right frame of mind)
Friday	£2 (didn't get enough sleep)
Saturday	£0 (nothing negative)
Sunday	£1 (googled IVF stats, which made me feel bad)
Total	£12

Closing balance for the week: £10
(opening balance of £7 plus income of £15 minus expenditure of £12)

We are most prone to stress overload when we have a lack of control over our circumstances and lack the resources to cope with those circumstances. This process will give you a sense of control and focus your mind on building resources to increase coping capacity. The following are some of the ways my clients say this technique has helped them.

I couldn't believe how much 'debt' I was in. No wonder the slightest little thing would tip me over the edge.

I felt empowered to make the right choices for myself. I was dreading my friend's baby shower, it was terrible timing for me. Normally I'd put myself through something like that at great emotional cost. But I could see from my 'bank balance' that I just couldn't afford to. Another time, maybe, but not right in the middle of my IVF cycle. My friend was fine and understood my decision.

I realised how rarely I do nice things for myself.

It was a wake-up call to see that everything I'd logged about my partner was negative. I knew I had to start investing in my relationship.

It helps me see how many good things I can make happen in my life.

I'd always thought the only way to reduce my stress was to stop doing certain things. It never occurred to me that I could reduce my overall stress load simply by looking after myself better and doing nice things.

A wellbeing bank account is much like an actual bank account. There are times when it's fine to go on a spending spree because you've built up a healthy bank balance. There are other times when a big expenditure plunges you into the red. This is just life. Some big expenditures are unexpected (like if the boiler breaks down), other times you plan and save up for them (like a holiday). When preparing for IVF, do all that you can to build up a nice healthy balance in your wellbeing bank account. That way you have plenty of 'cash' to spend when you need it.

7. Managing the 'two-week wait'

For the benefit of anyone who is unaware, the two-week wait (2WW) is the final stage of an IVF cycle – the bit after embryo transfer when you're waiting to take the pregnancy test. These days, the time period is often less than two weeks as clinics increasingly leave embryos to develop to blastocyst stage (for an explanation of all IVF stages please see chapter 2). The 2WW is frequently described as the most difficult part of IVF. Many of my clients begin working with me saying they are dreading it. But in my view the 2WW gets bad press. It really doesn't need to be so dreadful. It's my firm belief that if you've prepared well for IVF and created and maintained a healthy mindset it can be absolutely fine. It's probably not realistic to expect the best two weeks of your life – but it really can be OK.

All of the ideas presented in this chapter stand you in excellent stead for the 2WW. If you feel concerned about how you will cope at this time, or have had a difficult 2WW in the past, I encourage you to re-read the section on creating a healthy mindset (pages 59–68). As you do so, keep thoughts of the 2WW in mind and you will most likely find different things resonating for you. It will help you enormously to positively and purposely intend to cope well during your 2WW. And, of course, it is important to support that intention with healthy goals that help you to fill your days with activities that feel appropriate to you.

Some people find it helps to plan gentle activities to pass the time during their 2WW. Some set goals around things they never normally get around to, like sorting out photos, which can bring a satisfying sense of achievement. Others go on holiday. Some return to work and life as normal, or prefer to watch box sets. Different things are right for different people and any reputable fertility clinic will offer guidance on absolute dos and don'ts. So, I'm limiting myself to offering just one of each!

- Do make self-care your absolute priority during your 2WW.

- Don't view IVF as a series of stages to be successfully completed.

There are many stages to an IVF cycle (monitoring, down regulation, stimulation, egg retrieval, fertilisation, embryo transfer, waiting period and pregnancy test). However, it is not helpful to view each stage as something to be 'ticked off' before moving on to the next stage. This approach is unhelpful because you are in a constant state of waiting and uncertainty that causes the level of stress, anxiety, and anticipation to rise with each stage – peaking during the 2WW.

You are far more likely to experience a comfortable 2WW if, throughout your cycle, you stay present and focused on your intentions and goals – and you continue to apply this same level of focus throughout your 2WW.

As a final word on the 2WW, you may find it helpful to know that I rarely see clients during this period of their cycle. Most of my work involves creating a healthy mindset before IVF starts and then using mind-body techniques to enhance key stages of the cycle. After embryo transfer I keep an open slot in my diary, but I always leave it to the individual to contact me if they feel they need an appointment during their 2WW. In about 90 per cent of cases, I don't hear a word until after the pregnancy test. This is because they are fine and don't feel the need for extra support. The 2WW really can be OK.

8. Maintaining your relationship

For some couples, the realisation that starting a family is not going to be as simple as first believed can be the start of an emotional rollercoaster. Feelings of frustration, anger, blame, guilt, sadness and loss are not uncommon. Fun, laughter and enjoyment of intimacy can be forgotten after months or years of trying for a baby. IVF can put a strain on a relationship. But then again, pretty much anything – from back-seat driving to bankruptcy – can test a relationship if you let it. It's a question of mindset.

Everything that I've written so far is relevant to maintaining a healthy and loving relationship. If you feel that your relationship is under strain, I encourage you to re-read this chapter with your relationship in mind. Acknowledge what hurts, manage your expectations, intend for your relationship to thrive, take steps to manage your stress and invest in your relationship. These practical steps have the potential to reconnect you as friends, partners and lovers.

Many couples don't just survive IVF – they thrive. I am pleased to offer below a selection of suggestions, insights and experiences that may help you to do the same. Be mindful that your relationship is unique and not all 'good advice' is good for *you*. Apply your filter, notice what resonates and makes you stop and think about something a little differently.

- Be open about what each of you need – but be respectful and accepting of the fact that your needs may be very different. Intend to reach a mutually acceptable compromise.

- Don't set unreasonable privacy constraints. IVF is an emotional and sensitive topic. There may also be a whole host of personal, religious, cultural and professional reasons why people prefer to keep IVF a secret. But it's unreasonable to add the burden of complete secrecy to the already difficult process. For some people, sharing the ups and downs of IVF is an essential release. It can be very damaging to that person's mental wellbeing to enforce an absolute privacy rule. In all likelihood it will lead to many 'secret' conversations that begin with 'Don't tell my partner that I'm telling you this, but...' If privacy is very important to one of you, then compromise. Agree on one or two people 'the talker in the relationship' is allowed to share the journey with.

- Friends and family can be your best support or they can be your worst. Decide in advance who you will tell about IVF by identifying who will give you the support you need. In hindsight, many couples wish they had not told so many people at the start, as it sometimes adds to the pressure. Some couples find it helpful to designate a friend or family member as a 'spokesperson' who, when you are ready, will let others know what is going on. This can be particularly helpful on the day of your pregnancy test.

- Be open to the possibility that at times your partner may not be able to give you the support you need. Let that be OK. Accept that you may have a need that your partner simply isn't resourced to meet. Or perhaps isn't sufficiently resourced at that particular time. This doesn't mean your relationship is failing, this doesn't mean your partner doesn't care and this doesn't mean you must ignore your needs. Expecting your partner to be 'your everything' puts strain on a relationship. Sometimes a friend, parent, colleague or professional therapist is better placed to support you.

- Look outside your usual support network to those who truly understand what it is like to experience fertility problems. This may be a professional therapist, an online support group or a couple that you know have been through IVF. As always, apply your 'filter' in terms of what is useful and relevant for you as an individual and as a couple.

- Keep communicating throughout your fertility journey but place an agreed limit on fertility talk. Some couples find a limit of 20 minutes a day works for them. Some couples agree on times that are off-limits for fertility discussion, such as not within the first hour of getting home from work. It is important to agree on times to put fertility talk aside.

- Keep doing the things you enjoyed together as a couple before IVF.

- If your partner is experiencing side effects from the medication or is tired or upset, don't add to the burden by getting frustrated with her. Be kind. Let her know you appreciate what she is doing for you, your family and your future.

Note to the partner of a woman undergoing treatment: your partner needs you to support her emotionally every step of the way. She needs to feel like this is an equal priority for both of you and not something she has to deal with on her own. Take the time to explore and understand what she needs in terms of your support attending IVF appointments. Some couples agree that it is important to attend as many appointments together as possible, even after several failed cycles and the 'novelty' has worn off.

Some couples agree it's fine for the partner not undergoing treatment not to attend every IVF appointment. Listen for 'shoulds' and 'oughts' and stay present and true to YOUR needs and your relationship. Many women are perfectly happy to go to routine appointments such as blood tests on their own, and don't feel their partner 'should' be there. But note to the person not attending routine appointments: always call afterwards to find out how it went. It is important to let your partner know that you are just as invested in the results as she is.

Sadly, for some couples IVF may not result in the family they hoped for. But as an unknown author once said 'A bend in the road is not the end of the road… unless you fail to make the turn.' These couples will need strength from within, from each other and from others to enable them to make that turn. For other couples, when IVF brings a baby or babies, there is a whole new set of challenges and rewards waiting for the expectant parents. Irrespective of the outcome, many couples find the challenge of IVF improves their relationship and intimacy. Many couples find strengths and resources they had no idea were inside them. Many couples learn coping skills and communication patterns that provide life-long benefit. It will always be OK in the end. If it's not OK, it's not the end.

CHAPTER 4

Nutrition and IVF

Ms Neema Savvides BSc (Hons),
DipNT, mBANT

1. Introduction

Many couples overlook nutrition when it comes to their fertility, not realising just how much of an impact it can have on their ability to conceive. It is worth being mindful from the start that every cell in the body is affected by the foods that we eat. Therefore good-quality food equals good-quality egg and sperm cells too.

To help improve the chances of conception it is important to have the best-quality eggs and sperm in order to create the best-quality embryos. It can be useful to compare pre-IVF nutrition to studying for an exam – you wouldn't go into an exam unprepared, so why would you do the same with IVF? The best thing to do is to boost your chances by making sure you and your partner are in the best health, have the highest-quality eggs and sperm, and that your body has the right environment to aid embryo implantation and sustain a healthy pregnancy.

Unfortunately, most couples don't realise the importance of good nutrition until a failed first or second IVF cycle, then start searching for answers or explanations as to why their treatment didn't work.

Many people feel that conceiving should be straightforward, and yet it is not, for infertility rates are on the rise. While actual infertility rates are difficult to calculate, as there are so many potential factors that contribute to this, we do know that the number of people seeking and undergoing fertility treatment increased by 3.9 per cent from 2012 to 2013 (in 2013, 49,636 women had a total of 64,600 cycles of IVF or intra-cytoplasmic sperm injection (ICSI) and 2,379 women had a total of 4,611 cycles of donor insemination (DI). In 2012, 62,158 cycles of IVF or ICSI and 4,452 of DI were performed).[1] Further studies carried out by the HFEA report that the number of IVF cycles performed each year increased each year from 1991 to 2014.[2]

Good nutrition should be the first step on your IVF journey.

2. So where do you start?

It is recommended that both partners (male and female) address their fertility factors and start on a healthy nutritional plan at least sixty to ninety days prior to their IVF cycle in order to maximise their chances of success.

2.1 Why sixty to ninety days?

While we can improve upon the health and environment of our eggs, we need up to ninety days in order to do so. This is because the cycle of an egg in preparation for ovulation is ninety days, and it is within this time frame that the eggs are affected by both healthy and unhealthy factors.

3. Fertility factors to address

- Digestive health

- Stress

- Egg and sperm quality

- Toxic overload

- Hormonal imbalances

- Environment inflammation and blood flow to the uterus

- Hormone profile (FSH/AMH) – what this means and what you can do about it

4. Digestive health and why it's important

The core of any health concern starts with good digestive health. Without it, even the best diet in the world won't be truly effective.

The body needs to be able to digest the food consumed into forms it can then use, and thus be able to utilise the nutrients they provide. Essentially, with good digestive health and a comprehensive fertility diet, the body can then produce healthy sperm and eggs. On the flip side, if your gut is not functioning optimally then you are not digesting and absorbing enough nutrients. In order to make hormones, the body needs vitamins, minerals and nutrients. Very often in clinic clients present with digestive health issues, and it's no surprise given our modern-day lifestyles: high stress levels, convenience foods and poor diets.

4.1 What is poor digestion?

- Constipation

- Diarrhoea

- IBS (irritable bowel syndrome)

- Bloating

- Gas

- Heartburn

- Reflux

- Leaky gut

4.2 Signs of poor digestive health

- Bloating, belching, flatulence

- Fatigue, low iron levels

- Weak immune system (constantly feeling rundown and prone to illness)

- Weak and brittle nails

- Acne and other skin conditions such as eczema

- Food intolerances and allergies

- Inflammation

4.3 How to improve digestive health

- Avoid sugar.

- Eliminate any potential food sensitivities — wheat and dairy are common offenders. This is really important as these can affect digestion and will ultimately decrease your absorption of vital nutrients.

- Avoid processed foods.

- Increase fibre intake to encourage healthy bowel movements.

- Manage stress levels: exercise is a great stress reliever, as is meditation.

- Adopt an anti-inflammatory diet. Inflammation is part of the body's immune response and we need it in order to heal. However, when this response is out of control it can lead to conditions such as arthritis, migraines, obesity and cancer. Foods high in sugar and saturated fat trigger inflammation by causing overactivity in the immune system, leading to joint pain, fatigue and blood-vessel damage. Other foods such as oily fish help to curb inflammation.

- Take probiotics to boost beneficial bacteria in the gut.

- Take digestive enzymes. These tablets taken before meals help to break down the foods you eat into smaller components that the body can then absorb.

- Practise mindful eating. Eat away from any distractions such as the TV or your phone, chew your food thoroughly (20 times per bite) and take notice of the smells, tastes and textures of your food. Doing so encourages better digestion and the ability to recognise when you are full (not over-full).

5. Food intolerance vs food allergy

A food intolerance/sensitivity is different to a food allergy. A food allergy causes a specific and immediate immune response whereby the body interprets the food as harmful, and thus produces specific antibodies known as IgE antibodies to combat the food. These type of antibodies release histamines and other chemicals which can result in skin rashes or hives, breathing difficulties, swelling of the tongue and throat, anaphylactic shock, runny nose or abdominal pain. If you are allergic to a particular food it is important to avoid it. One of the most common allergens is peanuts.

A food intolerance/sensitivity, on the other hand, is caused by the body producing a different type of antibody known as an IgG antibody in response to the offending food item. This type of antibody produces a chronic inflammatory response resulting in damage to cells and tissues, and symptoms such as:

- Headaches

- Insomnia

- Fatigue

- Digestive problems such as constipation or flatulence

- Skin conditions such as acne

- Mood swings

- Sinus issues

- Weight gain/difficulty losing weight

- Muscle and joint pain

Many chronic health conditions can be attributed to inflammation such as:

- Migraines — inflammation of the blood vessels

- Arthritis — inflammation of the joints

- IBS — inflammation of the stomach and bowels which causes digestive disturbances

As the symptoms tend to be delayed (they appear anywhere from a few hours to a week) and can present in a combination, it is sometimes difficult to identify what the offending item is or even see the link between food consumption and symptoms.

6. How to tackle food intolerance

If you have been suffering from any of the above symptoms then you may have a food intolerance, although as there may be other underlying causes, always seek medical help. If you suspect a food intolerance/sensitivity the following can help you overcome these:

6.1 Identify your trigger foods

The most important thing to do is identify the trigger foods that are causing the inflammation. One way to do this is to conduct an elimination diet of the suspected offending foods or the most common offending foods (wheat, dairy, soy, additives, preservatives) for several days. Once this has been completed you can then introduce them back into your diet one at a time while noting down the symptoms.

Food intolerance testing, however, can be a much quicker and more accurate method of identifying possible trigger foods, and if you suspect you have a food intolerance this is a route you could take: find a reputable company like the London Allergy clinic or ask a qualified nutritional therapist to arrange the testing for you *as part of a* nutritional therapy consultation (contact BANT – the British Association for Nutrition and

Lifestyle Medicine, for a list of fully qualified nutritional therapists in your area).

6.2 Look for other hidden causes

Identifying food intolerances can be a tricky one as they can arise for a number and combination of different factors:

- A genuine intolerance where your body produces an inflammatory response.

- A digestive enzyme deficiency — Digestive enzymes are required to break down the food we eat into smaller components that the body is then able to use and absorb. Some people either lack the digestive enzyme(s) or do not have them in sufficient quantities. This can lead to incomplete digestion resulting in symptoms such as bloating, abdominal pain and flatulence. A common intolerance is a lactose intolerance whereby the sufferer does not have sufficient quantities of the enzyme lactase to break down lactose — the sugar found in milk products into smaller quantities that can then be absorbed by the gut. Undigested lactose is too large to be absorbed from the gut and its presence causes abdominal pain, bloating and diarrhoea. Imbalanced gut bacteria — a healthy balance of 'good' bacteria is required to keep the digestive system healthy. Any imbalance (caused by excess sugar intake, stress and inadequate nutrients to support the growth of good bacteria) in this can cause digestive disturbances. Consuming natural live yoghurt and taking a good-quality probiotic will help.

7. Digestion, inflammation and the effects on fertility

When the body detects something foreign such as chemicals, invading bacteria/viruses and pollen, the immune system sets out to attack it. This process is known as inflammation and is a specific immune response and is often due to the production of histamine. These small periods of inflammation are normal and designed to protect the body. However, sometimes inflammation can be present even without the presence of a foreign body, and this is when it can cause a problem. Many diseases and illnesses such as cancer, Alzheimer's, diabetes, arthritis, heart disease and depression have been linked to chronic inflammation.

One of the biggest effects of poor digestion is the inflammatory response it creates in the body. To put it simply, our bodies do not like inflammation. When inflammation is present, the body produces the stress hormone cortisol to compensate and help fight the inflammation. The presence of cortisol has an effect on important sex hormones such as the luteinising hormone (LH) and follicle-stimulating hormone (FSH), both of which affect fertility. From an IVF point of view, excessive inflammation may impact embryo implantation,[3] and exacerbate conditions such as PCOS, endometriosis, uterine fibroids and cysts, as well as contributing to recurrent miscarriages, anti-sperm antibodies, and Hashimoto's thyroiditis, an autoimmune disorder whereby the immune system attacks the body's own cells.

Issues such as IBS may suggest there is some form of inflammation in the body[4] (usually caused by food or chemical sensitivities), which result in a leaky gut, creating more inflammation. Leaky gut creates an environment where nutrients aren't being absorbed as much as they should be (which is also not ideal for pregnancy).

8. Anti-inflammatory diet

In order to reduce inflammation in your body it's important to remove any food sensitivities/intolerances that may be present in the diet. As already mentioned, wheat, dairy and sugar are common offenders. Include anti-inflammatory foods such as oats, oily fish and spices such as turmeric, and heal any damage caused to the digestive lining.

8.1 Inflammatory foods to avoid:

Food type	Example
Refined carbohydrates	White rice, white bread, cakes, sweets, chocolate
Red and processed meat	Steak, burgers, sausages
Sugary drinks	Fruit juice, squash, soft drinks, carbonated drinks
Processed and fried food	Crisps, chips, pizza

8.2 Anti-inflammatory foods to enjoy:

Food type	Good choices
Vegetables (organic if possible)	Spinach, kale, broccoli, carrots, cauliflower
Complex carbohydrates	Oats, quinoa, brown rice, legumes
Healthy fats	Olive oil, avocado, nuts (walnuts, Brazil nuts, almonds) seeds (flax, chia, pumpkin)
Fish and sea food	Wild salmon, mackerel, sardines
Fruit (organic if possible)	Raspberries, blueberries, strawberries, oranges
Spices	Garlic, turmeric, ginger, cinnamon

9. How good nutrition can help with stress

Good nutrition can help the body deal with the negative effects that stress places on it.

The body cannot distinguish between sources of stress, be they physical (actual physical danger, intensive exercise), emotional (work, bereavement, conceiving) or nutritional (the foods we eat such as caffeine, sugar and alcohol). When under stress, the body releases the hormone adrenaline to cope, which triggers the body's fight-or-flight response. This is helpful if we are in actual danger and need a boost of energy, quickened heart rate, sharpened vision, and thicker blood to help with wound healing. These are short-lived responses and once out of danger the body's nervous system returns to a less heightened state and hormone levels return to normal.

If, however, the source of the stress is mental or nutritional, these responses do not help. Being constantly stressed means the body is in this stress-responsive state for long periods of time, which leads to it prioritising the responses described above in favour of less urgent functions such as digestion (IBS in particular is exacerbated by stress).

10. How an improved diet can help with stress

In order to manage stress through diet, primarily you need to eat little and often, with each meal and snack containing a balance of protein, fat and carbohydrates. This helps to balance blood-sugar levels, which in turn manages stress and maintains energy levels.

10.1 Stress-busting nutrients:

- B vitamins. When stressed, our bodies consume B vitamins. As these are our energy vitamins, low levels can leave us feeling fatigued. Stock up on brown rice, quinoa, nuts, seeds, green leafy vegetables, meat and fish.

- Magnesium. Responsible for helping muscles to relax and reducing anxiety, magnesium is another nutrient that is depleted during stressful times. Brazil nuts are especially high in magnesium, as are brown rice, quinoa, oats, legumes and leafy green vegetables.

- Vitamin C. The adrenal glands help the body manage its stress response by producing stress hormones and contain the largest store of vitamin C. Increase your intake through oranges, kiwi, strawberries, tomatoes, peppers and green leafy vegetables. Low vitamin C levels decrease the activity of the immune cells that help fight bacteria and viruses, therefore keeping up your intake is especially important during times of stress. Zinc and vitamin A also help to boost the immune system and can be found in carrots, liver, oysters, pumpkin seeds and red meat. However once pregnant, care needs to be taken in relation to the amount of vitamin A consumed due to the fact that it is a fat-soluble vitamin and a build-up can be toxic to the foetus.

- Protein. During times of stress our bodies need more protein and inadequate intake can lead to poor immune function. Good sources include lean meats and poultry, eggs, pulses and oily fish like salmon and mackerel (these are especially good as they counteract the blood-thickening effects of adrenaline).

10.2 Stress-inducing substances to avoid:

- Caffeine. Found primarily in tea, coffee, energy drinks and chocolate, caffeine stimulates the adrenal glands to release the stress hormones described above. Avoid these if possible, or greatly reduce your intake, and switch to herbal teas and water. It's worth remembering that caffeine stays in your system for up to eight hours, so avoiding any after 2 p.m. will help you sleep better. Good-quality sleep is crucial to managing stress levels.

- Sugar, salt, alcohol and nicotine. These stimulate the body's stress response and deplete the body of essential nutrients.

11. How can we balance hormones?

- Managing sugar levels by eating small meals throughout the day, and being aware of sugar intake

- Consuming healthy fats (found in avocados, nuts such as Brazil, walnuts, almonds; seeds like pumpkin, flax, chia and sunflower)

- Supporting digestive health by managing sugar intake and eating gut-friendly foods such as oats and oily fish

12. Obesity and how it can affect IVF success

Body mass index (BMI) is a measure of body weight based upon height and weight. It's a useful tool to estimate the optimal body weight for your height and is calculated using the formula below. Your BMI will indicate whether you are at a normal/healthy weight, underweight, overweight or obese (table below). *Please note these are the guidelines for adults only.*

BMI = weight in kg/height in metres squared

BMI results

18.5 or less	Underweight
18.5–24.9	Normal
25.0–29.9	Overweight
30.0–34.9	Obese
35.5 – 39.9	Obese
40 +	Extremely obese

A study carried out by Guy's and St Thomas' NHS Foundation Trust has shown that being overweight (and not just obese) can affect IVF success.[5] This study of 400 women between 2006 and 2010 showed that women with a BMI of 25 or over had double the miscarriage risk compared to women with a normal BMI – that is 38 versus 20. The miscarriage rates between the overweight and obese groups were 37 and 42 respectively, showing a 5 increase between the two. One of the reasons for this could be due to increased levels of the hormones insulin and leptin in overweight women, which affect the lining of the womb (endometrium) and thus implantation of the embryo.

The recommendation based upon this study is that women come as close to a normal/healthy weight as soon as possible prior to treatment in order to maximise their chances of IVF success.

It is also thought that obese women have diminished IVF success due to poorer egg quality and are likely to have reduced IVF success and poorer reproductive health in general.

13. Good nutrition and how it can help you achieve a healthy/normal weight, ideal for IVF

Weight loss is so much more than 'calories in vs calories out' and it's definitely not 'one size fits all'. Some of the best and easiest weight-loss guidance includes the following:

- Eat balanced meals. Ensure each meal has a balance of protein (poultry, fish, meat, beans and pulses), complex carbohydrates (sweet potatoes, oats, brown rice, quinoa) and healthy fats (avocado, olive/coconut oil).

- Eat until satisfied, not full. This is a difficult one to master but stopping when you are 7/10 satisfied on the hunger scale will help you to not overeat.

- Eat slowly, eat mindfully and chew your food thoroughly. It takes 20 minutes for the brain to register that the stomach is full.

- Watch your portion sizes. If you look at your plate aim for half of it being green leafy vegetables, a quarter protein and a quarter carbohydrates.

- Don't drink your calories — this includes soft drinks, fruit juices, flavoured coffees etc

- Eliminate processed and sugary foods. This is generally most things that come out of a packet (ready meals, crisps, biscuits, chocolates, etc.).

- Reduce carbohydrate intake in the evenings.

- Stay hydrated! Most people overeat when they are actually thirsty. Aim for at least 2 litres of filtered water per day.

- Keep moving! Find an activity you love and keep at it.

14. Good nutrition and how it can boost egg quantity and quality

Egg health is one of the cornerstones of fertility. The health of your eggs may well determine whether or not fertilisation and implantation will occur as well as whether the pregnancy will be viable.

Women are born with all of the egg cells that we have for the rest of our lives, which is why age has such an impact on egg health and the number of eggs we have (ovarian reserve). As we age, the ovaries age, making the environment for the eggs less than optimal. Therefore it's essential to protect ovarian reserve through diet, supplements and making the most beneficial lifestyle choices.

15. Hormones – FSH and AMH

Ovarian reserve describes the current supply of eggs a woman has within her ovaries. It is determined by the hormonal panels FSH (follicular-stimulating hormone) and AMH (anti-Müllerian hormone)

If you have high FSH levels and low AMH, this can indicate ovaries that are not responding well to IVF medications, poor-quality eggs and diminishing ovarian reserve. It's important therefore to be aware of all factors that can be an improvement to the health of your eggs.

16. Factors contributing to good egg health

16.1 Blood flow and circulation

We need good circulation to distribute oxygen and nutrient -rich blood to our ovaries and throughout our systems to keep us healthy and feeling energised. Good circulation removes toxins and lactic acid, brings blood to our muscles, keeps our brain focused and brings colour to our skin.

Our modern-day lifestyles mean we spend more time sitting at our desks, watching TV or in the car than we used to. Our circulation becomes sluggish as a result, which means it's even more important to get our blood moving properly. We need oxygen and nutrient-rich blood to flow properly to the ovaries. This can be achieved by employing the following lifestyle changes:

16.2 Get moving

Physical activity is by far the best way of improving circulation. By getting the heart pumping and the circulatory system moving we help to oxygenate the blood, and increase the flow of fresh blood, which brings oxygen and nutrients to the reproductive cells. Any movement is better than none, so find something you enjoy and stick to it, whether it's walking, chasing the dog or group sports and activities. If you have a desk job remember to stand up and have a walk around at least every hour to get your body moving. This doesn't have to be strenuous – a simple walk to get some water or to speak to a colleague will suffice.

16.3 Drink at least 2 to 3 litres of pure/filtered water per day

When you are dehydrated your blood thickens, which slows down circulation and causes many other issues. Make sure you avoid water in plastic bottles though, as plastic is thought to affect our hormones. Plastics are made from chemicals called xenohormones which are thought to mimic hormones and disrupt the way hormones are produced, metabolised and eliminated from the body, thereby disrupting our hormonal balance.[6]

16.4 Consume iron-rich foods and citrus fruits

Both of these have been found to improve circulation, and consuming citrus fruits (oranges, kiwis, limes) with iron-rich foods helps the body to absorb the iron (found in red meat, green leafy vegetables, beans and pulses).

16.5 Balance your hormones

If your hormones are out of balance, your eggs may not respond properly to the fertility medications. Our entire reproductive system is governed by our hormones, and problems can occur when there is too little or too much oestrogen, too little progesterone, excessive male hormones, and high or low levels of cortisol (stress hormones).

We are often stressed and overworked, and grab easy food on the go. This is low in nutritional value and contains high amounts of trans-fatty acids, which are considered to be the worst kind of fats to eat, especially for fertility; they also raise bad (LDL) cholesterol and lower good (HDL) cholesterol.

It's essential to eat well and maintain a healthy body weight in order to support the hormonal functioning in your body, so as to maximise your chances of conception.

17. Diet, digestive function and hormones

Your nutritional status and digestive function are the two components that determine how well your hormones will be balanced, and thus determine your fertility levels. This is because hormones require specific nutrients to be healthy, such as essential fatty acids, vitamins A and B6, zinc, magnesium and antioxidants. Digestive function is crucial when our body, burdened with sugar, fatty and processed foods, has to use valuable energy (that could have been utilised for reproduction) to process them. The body and liver then have to work at detoxifying, rather than reproducing. Once hormones are used, they are processed by the liver and passed to the digestive system to be eliminated. By overburdening the liver and digestive systems we cannot clear excess hormones efficiently, which leads to a build-up in the body. This is why I always recommend some form of liver cleanse prior to commencing fertility treatment.

18. Weight and hormones

Earlier in the chapter we discussed the effects of obesity on conception. We now know that our fat cells continually release oestrogen which can affect our hormonal balance. The more fat cells you have, the more oestrogen gets released. High levels of oestrogen can also affect FSH levels and ovarian reserve.

Being underweight is just as much of a concern as it can

cause oestrogen levels to drop, affecting menstruation and the quality of cervical mucus. If you do become pregnant while underweight it can lead to risks such as premature births and low birth weight. Eating well and gaining sufficient weight to ensure you are within a healthy weight range can help.

19. Nutrition and hormones

As discussed previously, during this 90-day period what you eat can impact the health of your eggs and ovaries, either positively or negatively. Good-quality eggs are born from a nutritionally dense diet.

19.1 Key nutrients for egg health

Nutrient	How it helps	Good sources
Vitamin D	Helps the body to create sex hormones, which in turn affect ovulation and hormonal balance.	Oily fish, fortified eggs, cod liver oil and sunlight.
Antioxidants	Vitamins A, C, E, zinc, selenium and CoQ10 are powerful antioxidants and help to protect eggs from damage caused by free radicals so consuming antioxidant-rich foods is vital to protect the eggs.	Berries, peppers, green leafy vegetables and nuts such as almonds.

Nutrient	How it helps	Good sources
Amino acids / L-arginine	Amino acids are the building blocks of every cell in the body, thus they are crucial for reproductive health. The amino acid L-arginine in particular is important to help boost ovarian response, endometrial receptivity and blood circulation which helps to transport oxygen and nutrients to the reproductive system.	Walnuts, Brazil nuts and seafood. Lean meat, fish, poultry, legumes walnuts, Brazil nuts and seafood.
Essential fatty acids	These help to regulate hormones, increase cervical mucus, promote ovulation, increase blood flow to the uterus (thus boosting its health) and help to reduce inflammation.	Aim to consume salmon, mackerel or sardines two or three times a week. Flax seeds, walnuts and chia seeds are also good sources.
Zinc	As well as being an antioxidant, zinc is a key nutrient used in over 300 enzyme reactions in the body. Without it, your cells can't divide properly and your hormones	Oysters, lean red meat, poultry, pumpkin and sunflower seeds, eggs and pulses.

Nutrient	How it helps	Good sources
	(oestrogen and progesterone) get out of balance. Low levels of zinc have been linked to miscarriages in the early stages of pregnancy.	
Iron	Low iron levels can result in a lack of ovulation and poor egg health, which can affect your chances of conceiving.	Lean red meat, spinach, lentils, pumpkin and sesame seeds.
Vitamin B6	This is an important hormone regulator, eases PMS and helps to regulate blood sugar levels.	Tuna, bananas, turkey, salmon, brightly coloured and green vegetables.
Vitamin B12	This important vitamin helps to boost the endometrium lining, thus reducing the chances of miscarriage.	Oysters, lobster, beef, lamb and eggs.
Folic acid	Folic acid helps to prevent neural tube defects.	Liver, lentils, asparagus and kidney beans.

19.2 Foods to avoid

Avoid sugar, alcohol and caffeine, which disrupt hormones. They place a burden on the liver, forcing it to work harder and thus take away focus from hormone regulation, which is needed to produce healthy eggs.

Avoid non-organic meat and dairy, which are high in hormones and antibiotics, which can affect ovulation.

19.3 Toxin exposure

Limit exposure to toxins as they can affect the health of the egg. Toxins can be found in unfiltered tap and bottled water, pesticides, sugar (bread, pasta, noodles, cakes, chocolate and biscuits), processed foods (ready meals, breakfast bars), non-organic meat, dairy and caffeine. Reducing your caffeine and sugar intakes will help, as will consuming organic foods and drinking filtered water/ water in glass bottles. Ideally try to consume natural foods – avoid anything processed.

Constipation can lead to a build-up of toxins so it's important to encourage regular bowel movements by eating a high-fibre diet.

To combat toxin exposure it is also important to consume a wide variety of antioxidant-rich foods. These are found in berries, green leafy vegetables (broccoli, spinach, cabbage), peppers, carrots and essentially any brightly coloured fruits or vegetables, as well as oily fish salmon, mackerel and sardines.

Water is key as it helps to remove toxins, increases blood flow and is needed for proper digestion. Aim for 1.5 to 2 litres a day.

20. Sperm quality and morphology

The shape of sperm is an important factor in determining whether or not it is able to fertilise an egg. The egg has a protein coat, and its first function is to decide which sperm will fertilise the egg. The sperm therefore need to be super motile and the sperm head needs to be the correct shape and size (symmetrical and oval) in order to penetrate the egg's outer shell. Poor morphology means that sperm are irregularly shaped, too long, too short, too round, too big or too small. The egg will then prevent these from penetrating the outer shell and thus fertilisation cannot occur.

The biggest factors affecting morphology are genetics, toxin exposure and increased testicular temperature.

20.1 Key nutrients to boost sperm quality and quantity

Nutrient	How it helps	Good sources
Amino acids	These protein building blocks help to boost sperm quantity and the amino acid L-arginine is especially important and can help to boost blood circulation.	Walnuts, Brazil nuts and seafood. Supplements can also be beneficial.
Essential fatty acids	Sperm contain large amounts of DHA, the omega-3 fatty acid, with the majority being found in the tail, so omega-3s are vital for sperm motility.	Aim to consume salmon, mackerel and sardines two or three times a week.
Antioxidants	Free-oxidising radicals can cause sperm damage so a diet rich in vitamins A, C, E, zinc and selenium is vital to protect the sperm, reduce clumping, abnormalities and increase motility.	Berries, peppers, green leafy vegetables and nuts such as almonds.
Zinc	As well as being an antioxidant, zinc is a key nutrient for the production of healthy sperm, boosting	Pumpkin and sun-flower seeds, lean meat and poultry, eggs and pulses can help to replenish stores.

Nutrient	How it helps	Good sources
	motility, and helping to remove excess oestrogen from the body (high levels of which is linked to low sperm count), and is commonly lacking is most people's diets. Zinc is lost through ejaculation so consuming zinc-rich foods is important to replenish stores.	
CQ10	This is a powerful antioxidant helping to protect the sperm and increase its motility.	Seafood and organ meats.
Vitamin B12	This important vitamin can help to increase sperm count, due to its role in duplicating DNA in cells, increasing metabolism and providing energy and resources to manufacture new sperm cells.	Oysters, lobster, beef, lamb and eggs.
Folic acid	Helps to boost sperm health.	Liver, lentils, asparagus and kidney beans.

Toxins can affect sperm quality and can be found in cigarette smoke, alcohol, pesticides, sugar (bread, pasta, noodles, cakes, chocolate, biscuits), processed foods (ready meals, bacon and sausages), caffeine, tap and bottled water. These toxins force the liver to work harder which takes the focus away from its role in hormone regulation, which is needed to produce healthy sperm. Reducing your smoking, alcohol, caffeine and sugar intakes will help, as will consuming organic foods and drinking filtered water/ water in glass bottles. Ideally you want to consume natural foods so avoid anything processed.

Prolonged sitting and wearing tight clothing mean that the testicles are drawn closer to the body, increasing their temperature. Sperm prefer cooler temperatures, which is why the testicles drop from the body. Getting up and walking around every so often and wearing loose underwear can help.

When boosting sperm health, it's important to ensure that male hormones are balanced. Imbalanced hormones are caused by oestrogen-mimicking foods which lower fertility-boosting testosterone. High oestrogen levels can lead to erectile dysfunction and a decreased sperm count, libido and seminal fluid.

Oestrogen can be found in soy products, pesticides in fruits and vegetables, hormones in meat and dairy, and plastics so it is vital to consume organic produce, drink filtered water from glass bottles, avoid heating plastics (like Tupperware or soup containers).

In addition a high-fibre and liver-supporting diet

is crucial to help the body clear any excess hormones. Increase your intake of green leafy vegetables, quinoa, sweet potatoes, pumpkin, sunflower and sesame seeds.

Zinc, selenium, omega-3s, antioxidants and folic acid are crucial for sperm health and these can be found in Brazil nuts, pumpkin and sunflower seeds, eggs, lean meat and poultry, oily fish, brightly coloured fruits and vegetables and dark green leafy vegetables.

21. Liver Detox

21.1 Pre IVF liver detox (for both women and men)

The liver plays an important role in the body, from managing and processing toxins to processing of hormones, so it's essential to keep it healthy. This is especially important if you have a previous failed IVF cycle or used fertility drugs, where there will be excess hormone levels in your body. Fertility drugs can also have side effects and be toxic, so it's important to follow a cleanse specifically designed for preconception to boost uterine health.

Men who smoke can find a detox extremely beneficial as smokers tend to have lower sperm counts, poor motility and higher morphology rates (abnormal sperm). By embarking on a detox we can ensure healthier sperm cells are produced.

This detox is designed to help clear your body of excess hormones and toxins, as well as improving circulation to your reproductive system in preparation for IVF.

21.2 Benefits of a liver detox:

- It supports the liver, thereby encouraging its detoxification process

- It helps to eliminate excess hormones that can affect fertility and conception

- It can eliminate old, stagnant blood, clots and debris, thereby creating the right environment for conception

- It can help reduce inflammation of the reproductive organs

- It increases circulation of fresh oxygenated blood to the reproductive area

21.3 Toxin reduction

During this detox it is important to avoid the following toxins:

To be avoided	Examples
Caffeine	Tea, coffee, energy drinks, soft drinks (cola, carbonated drinks)
Alcohol	Wine, beer, spirits
Cigarettes	
Refined sugars	Sweets, cakes, biscuits, chocolate, soft drinks
Saturated fats	Red meat
Wheat, gluten, yeast	Bread, pasta, noodles
Dairy	Milk, cheese, yoghurt
Processed foods	Ready meals, crisps
Spreads	Jam, chocolate, peanut butter
Artificially produced flavourings	Ketchup, vinegar, mustard

21.4 The Liver Detox Plan

Day	Upon rising	Breakfast	Snack	Lunch	Dinner	Snack
1	Cup of hot water and lemon + probiotic	Liver detox juice	Herbal tea	Blueberry and almond milk smoothie	Detox green soup	10 almonds and a cup of dandelion tea
2	Cup of hot water and lemon + probiotic	Raspberry and almond milk smoothie (follow recipe for blueberry smoothie, replacing blueberries with raspberries)	Liver detox juice	Raw avocado and tomato soup	Detox green soup	Herbal tea
3	Cup of hot water and lemon + probiotic	Beetroot, carrot, apple and ginger juice	5 Brazil nuts	Raw kale salad with avocado and tomato	Spinach soup	Herbal tea
4	Cup of hot water and lemon + probiotic	Beetroot, carrot, apple and ginger juice	5 walnuts and a cup of dandelion tea	Blueberry and almond milk smoothie	Detox green soup	Herbal tea

5	Cup of hot water and lemon + probiotic	Blueberry, banana and almond milk smoothie (follow recipe for blueberry and almond milk smoothie and add a small banana)	Dandelion tea	Cucumber and avocado soup	Detox green soup	5 Brazil nuts and herbal tea
6	Cup of hot water and lemon + probiotic	Beetroot, carrot, apple and ginger juice	10 almonds	Raw kale salad with avocado and tomato	Baked wild salmon with spinach	Herbal tea
7	Cup of hot water and lemon + probiotic	3 tablespoons of natural yoghurt topped with cinnamon, flaxseeds, toasted pumpkin and sesame seeds half-cup of blueberries and half-cup raspberries	Herbal tea	Omelette (organic eggs) made with peppers, onions, mushrooms and broccoli	Cucumber and avocado soup	5 walnuts and herbal tea

22. Detox recipes

(Be sure to use organic produce for all the recipes.)

LIVER DETOX JUICE

Serves: 1

(If you are on prescription medications, please make sure you check the contraindications of grapefruit with your GP, as grapefruit can have harmful effects if taken with certain medications. Substitute with blood oranges if required.)

Ingredients
1 large grapefruit
2 lemons
20 ml (1 cup) filtered water
2 tablespoons cold-pressed flax oil/extra virgin olive oil
1–2 cloves of fresh garlic, peeled
5cm (2 inches) fresh root ginger, peeled
2 tablespoons cold-pressed flax oil/extra virgin olive oil
Optional: a dash of cayenne pepper

Directions

Squeeze the juice of the grapefruit and lemon into a blender.

Grate the garlic and the ginger, and then using a garlic press, squeeze this into the juice.

Add the water and oil; blend for 30 seconds.

Add more ginger and/or garlic to taste, and a dash of cayenne pepper if desired.

This juice contains all of the most potent liver-cleansing ingredients, and gives your liver a gentle flush and the opportunity to heal itself. There are no side effects to this drink, apart from a bit of garlic breath for a while. However, the grapefruit removes most of the odour.

BLUEBERRY AND ALMOND MILK SMOOTHIE

Serves: 1

Ingredients
2 tablespoons hemp/brown rice protein powder
75g (½ cup) blueberries
1 scoop greens powder (optional)
1 tablespoon flax seeds
350ml (1½ cup) almond milk

Directions
Blend everything together
Feel free to substitute the almond milk with coconut milk

DETOX GREEN SOUP

Serves: 2

The consistency of this easy detox soup can be changed to suit personal taste by adjusting the amount of water that you add to it.

Ingredients
1 tablespoon olive oil
2 cloves of garlic, chopped
2 tablespoons diced onion
1 inch of fresh ginger, peeled and chopped
300g (4 cups) fresh broccoli, cut up small
225g (½lb) fresh spinach leaves
3 parsnips, peeled, cored, chopped
2 sticks celery, trimmed, chopped
Handful of fresh parsley, roughly chopped
Fresh water, as needed
Sea salt and ground pepper, to taste
Lemon or lime juice

Directions
Using a large soup pot, heat the olive oil over medium heat and stir in the garlic, onion, and ginger to season the oil. Add the broccoli, spinach, parsnips, celery and parsley, and stir until the

spinach wilts and collapses. Add just enough water to cover the vegetables. Remember the spinach will cook down quite a bit, so don't add too much water at first. You can always thin the soup later, if required.

Bring to a high simmer, cover the pot, and reduce the heat to a medium simmer. Cook for 15 minutes or until the vegetables have softened.

Use a blender/hand blender to purée the soup.

Season with salt and pepper and add a squeeze of lemon if it needs brightening.

Option: To make this into a creamy soup add a dash of coconut milk.

RAW AVOCADO AND TOMATO SOUP

Serves: 2

Ingredients
3 ripe avocados
3 tomatoes
2 handfuls of fresh spinach
2 teaspoons freshly squeezed lemon juice
A pinch of Himalayan crystal salt or Celtic sea salt

Freshly ground pepper
A small amount of water (depending on how liquid you like the soup to be)

Directions
Cut the tomatoes into small pieces.
Put all the ingredients except the tomato pieces into a mixer. Mix well on the highest setting.
Pour the soup into a soup bowl and add the tomato pieces.

BEETROOT, CARROT, APPLE AND GINGER JUICE

Serves: 1

Ingredients
1 large or 2 medium beetroots, cut into wedges
½ lemon, zest and pith removed
2 large carrots
1 large apple, cut into wedges
2.5 cm (1inch) length of ginger

Directions
Juice everything into a glass, stir and enjoy!

RAW KALE, AVOCADO AND TOMATO SALAD

Serves: 2

Ingredients
One large bunch of kale
1½ tablespoons extra virgin olive oil
½ avocado, peeled and chopped
1 'heirloom' (or 'heritage') tomato, chopped
1 teaspoon freshly grated ginger
2 tablespoons roasted sunflower seeds
Juice from half of a lemon or lime
Sea salt and pepper

Directions
Wash and dry the kale thoroughly. Remove the stems from the kale leaves and rip or chop the leaves into bite-sized pieces. Put these into a large bowl and add the olive oil. Massage the oil into the kale leaves until they are fully coated. Add in a pinch of salt and the avocado pieces. Massage the kale leaves again until they are fully coated. Work the avocado in. Set aside to marinate for 15 minutes.

Add lemon or lime juice, chopped tomato, grated ginger and sunflower seeds. Toss and season with salt and pepper to taste. Eat and enjoy!

SPINACH SOUP

Serves: 2

Spinach is full of iron, vitamins and calcium; it is also essential fibre. Care should be taken that the vegetables are organic because they are grown without using herbicides, fertilisers or pesticides, all containing toxins that would cancel the benefits of the diet.

Ingredients
2 tablespoons cold-pressed olive oil
1 teaspoon chopped garlic
125g (1 cup) diced leek
125g (1 cup) diced celery
125g (1 cup) diced carrots
150g (1 cup) diced onion
600ml (6 cups) of water
2 bay leaves
1 sprig thyme
900g (2lb) chopped spinach

Directions
In a large pot, sauté the garlic in the olive oil for two minutes and then add the leek, celery, carrots and onion. Cook until the onions appear translucent, then add water, bay leaves and thyme.

Bring to the boil and then reduce the heat, cover and let it simmer for one hour. Take the pot off the heat and leave to cool for another hour; strain out the bay leaves and thyme.

Take this mixture and make a purée of it in a blender or food processor, then add the spinach to it and cook the soup over a medium heat until the spinach has wilted. Be careful not to overcook the spinach as it destroys its nutritional value.

CUCUMBER AND AVOCADO SOUP

Serves: 1

Ingredients
3 avocados, stone removed and chopped up
Zest of ½ lime
Juice of 1 lime
½ teaspoon salt
1 cucumber, peeled and seeded, roughly chopped

Directions
Blend all the ingredients together until totally creamy and smooth.

BAKED SALMON WITH SPINACH

Serves: 1

Ingredients
1 organic salmon fillet
1 clove garlic, minced
½ chilli pepper
2.5 cm (1inch) grated ginger
½ a lemon
Freshly ground black pepper to taste
Handful chopped coriander
60g (2 cups) spinach

Directions
Place salmon in the middle of a large piece of foil.
Top with garlic, chilli, ginger and coriander and
squeeze of lemon. Add pepper to taste. Bake in the
oven (190/gas mark 5) for 15 minutes. Serve on a
bed of wilted spinach.

23. Pre-IVF diet plan

This prepares and supports your body in its reproductive efforts. The general plan that follows covers those foods to avoid or reduce and those you can enjoy to your heart's content, as well as giving a number of meal and snack suggestions.

23.1 Foods to avoid/reduce

- Caffeine
- Alcohol
- Non-organic meats
- Farmed fish
- Sugar
- Soft drinks
- Soya — soya milk, tofu, etc.
- Processed foods and meats (crisps, ready meals, sausages, salami, etc.)
- Refined sugars (bread, pasta, cakes, biscuits, white rice)
- Tap water
- Wheat (and gluten)

23.2 Foods to enjoy

(and the vitamins, minerals and other nutrients they provide)

- Organic eggs: protein, vitamins D, B12

- Nuts and seeds (especially pumpkin, sesame, walnuts, almonds, Brazil nuts): omega-3, zinc, vitamin E, protein, selenium

- Organic dark leafy green vegetables (spinach, broccoli, kale, etc.): Iron, folic acid, vitamins B6 and E, fibre

- Berries (blueberries, raspberries, strawberries): vitamin C (antioxidants), flavonoids

- Grass-fed/organic meat and poultry: protein, omega-3, iron, vitamin B12

- Wild-caught fish — aim for two portions of oily fish per week (salmon, mackerel, sardines)

- Organic colourful vegetables: vitamin B6, antioxidants

- Lentils and beans: iron, folic acid, protein

- Low-GI carbohydrates (sweet potato, butternut squash, quinoa, brown rice): vitamins C and A, magnesium, fibre

- Filtered water — at least 2 litres a day

Note: Remember to include some form of protein in every meal and snack. This is very important, especially during the egg stimulation stage of your IVF cycle as it can really boost your response.

23.3 Breakfast ideas

- Smoothie made with almond milk, 1 scoop protein powder, 5 Brazil nuts, large handful of spinach/kale, handful of berries, ½ banana, 1 tablespoon flax seeds and a sprinkling of cinnamon. You can add 1 to 2 teaspoons of spirulina powder to this.

- Green smoothie made with 1 scoop protein powder (e.g. Vega Sport), 2.5cm (1 inch) ginger, ¼ cucumber, 1 stick celery, squeeze of lime/lemon, ½ frozen banana, 5 Brazil nuts.

- Quinoa porridge.

- Porridge made with almond milk, topped with nuts, flaxseeds and berries.

- Muesli — soak oats/quinoa flakes in almond milk, nuts, seeds and cinnamon, top with berries in the morning (you can make a large batch of this and store it in the fridge for up to 5 days).

- Omelette made with spinach, tomatoes and peppers served with rye bread (optional).

- Organic live yoghurt topped with ½ banana, cinnamon, berries, flaxseeds and sunflower seeds.

- Scrambled eggs on rye (occasionally only, as rye bread contains wheat) with a side of spinach, tomatoes and half an avocado.

23.4 Lunch ideas

- Homemade soup – vegetable or vegetable-based; preferably chicken or lentil. If buying soup, buy organic. Avoid heating the soup in its plastic container (transfer to a glass bowl instead).

- 2-egg frittata made with 5 to 6 large handfuls of baby spinach, diced sweet potato and tomato. Top with ½ sliced avocado.

- Mackerel with butternut squash and broccoli.

- If buying ready-made salads, look for something containing protein, colourful vegetables and either quinoa or root vegetables.

23.5 Dinner ideas

- Beef stir-fry (strips of beef with onions, carrots, cabbage, broccoli and peppers cooked in olive oil and flavoured with garlic, chilli and ginger).

- Fishcakes made with salmon, haddock and sweet potato served with spinach/asparagus.

- Salmon with a walnut crust (crush walnuts and place on top of a piece of cooked salmon), served with broccoli.

- Mixed roasted Mediterranean vegetables served with grilled white fish.
- Lamb/chicken/beef/prawn curry (mix in spinach/kale) served with a small portion of brown rice/quinoa.
- Grilled chicken with a side of roasted cauliflower.
- Quinoa with roasted vegetables topped with pine nuts.

23.6 Snack ideas

- Crudités (mixed raw vegetables) with organic hummus
- Crudités with guacamole
- Piece of fruit (apple/pear) and 5 almonds/Brazil nuts/walnuts
- Rye bread spread with pumpkin seed/almond butter (available from most supermarkets/health food shops)
- Smoked mackerel pâté (make with organic Greek yoghurt instead of cream cheese) with celery/cucumber
- Coconut pieces
- Sashimi

24. Nutrition goals post-embryo transfer

- Increase antioxidant intake (green leafy vegetables, brightly coloured fruits and vegetables).
- Increase protein intake — lean meat and fish, beans and pulses.

- High anti-inflammatory diet — oats, fish, avocados, nuts, seeds, vegetables.

- Water intake — at least 2 litres per day.

- Stick to organic foods where possible.

24.1 Foods to avoid post-embryo transfer

- Caffeine — try rooibos tea, which is caffeine free and full of antioxidants

- Alcohol

- Sugar, wheat, carbonated drinks, processed food

- Tuna (high in mercury)

- Processed and packaged foods

- Raw fish (sushi/sashimi)

- Pâté

- Fatty, heavy and spicy foods (fine to eat curry but reduce the amount of chilli used)

25. Conclusion

In this chapter, we've discussed how optimising your nutrition can increase your chances of IVF success. Ideally, a couple will start to optimise their nutrition at least ninety days prior to starting an IVF cycle. However, if you're reading this and your IVF cycle is due to start in less than ninety days please be assured that any improvements you can make to your diet and lifestyle will be of benefit.

Within this chapter, I've outlined the many fertility factors that good nutrition can assist with: digestive health, balancing hormones, achieving a normal/healthy BMI, stress, egg and sperm quality. We've talked about the benefits of a pre-IVF liver detox and how following a pre-IVF diet plan can ensure you're consuming the most beneficial foods and avoiding foods that cause inflammation and hormonal imbalance.

I hope this chapter has demonstrated the important role that nutrition can play on your IVF journey.

References

1. HFEA Fertility Trends and Figures 2013; http://www.hfea.gov.uk/docs/HFEA_Fertility_Trends_and_Figures_2013.pdf.

2. HFEA Fertility Treatment and Trends Figures 2014; http://www.hfea.gov.uk/docs/HFEA_Fertility_treatment_Trends_and_figures_2014.pdf.

3. http://www.ncbi.nlm.nih.gov/pmc/articles/PMC3025807/.

4. Liebregts, T., Birgit, A., Bredack, C., Roth, et al., 'Immune Activation in Patients with Irritable Bowel Syndrome', *Gastroenterology*, 2007, 132:913–920; http://www.gastrojournal.org/article/S0016-5085(07)00185-0/abstract.

5. http://humrep.oxfordjournals.org/content/26/10/2642.

6. Yang, C. Z., Yaniger, S. I., Jordan, V. Craig, Study: 'Most Plastic Products Release Estrogenic Chemicals: A Potential Health Problem That Can Be Solved'; http://www.ncbi.nlm.nih.gov/pmc/articles/PMC3222987/.

CHAPTER 5

Embryo Quality and Factors Affecting It

Christine Leary, BSc, HCPC, FRCPath, PhD, Consultant
Embryologist and Director at the Hull IVF Unit

1. Introduction

One of the biggest challenges for any IVF clinic and specifically any embryologist, is choosing which embryo to transfer and explaining why one embryo, would be favoured over another and what the embryo grading score assigned actually means to you, the patient. Whether you are attempting IVF treatment for the first time or trying to understand what factors may have contributed to your embryo quality and a previous treatment outcome, this chapter will aim to explain how an embryo's potential to form a baby is determined. There is compelling evidence in the scientific literature to suggest that embryo developmental quality is highly predictive of IVF cycle outcome; however, the factors predisposing an embryo to arrest its development are largely predetermined before the egg and sperm meet to form the embryo. This implies that the egg and sperm quality and the maternal/ paternal environment from which they are derived i.e. your general health and lifestyle, are fundamental to your reproductive success.

2. Embryo quality

During an IVF treatment cycle you will hear lots about embryo quality/ embryo grading and development. Embryo quality is graded at various points of development, and numerous markers of an embryo's viability and ability to implant have been identified. Historically, embryos are first graded on day 2 and day 3 of development, at the 'cleavage stage' and at this point, graded according to their cell number and the appearance of these cells (their morphology).

The embryo cell (sometimes called blastomere) number, should be appropriate for the time of assessment (i.e. if you are discussing your embryo development two days after egg collection, you would be hoping to hear that your embryos had reached 2–4 cells and likewise if on day 3 of development hopefully the embryos will be at the 6–8 cell stage), with slow-growing and unusually fast-growing embryos being less likely to implant and possibly more likely to contain chromosome abnormalities. Observations are also recorded on the appearance (morphology) of the cells of the embryo, and those containing lots of fragmented or uneven cells are deemed to be of lower quality. Fragments may occur when a cell divides, similar to when you break a square of chocolate in half you may not get a clean or even break. Generally, the embryos are then scored from 1 to 4, denoting low to high quality.

While these observations and grading assessment criteria may be subjective and imprecise, it has been consistently shown that embryos with higher fragmentation are less likely to implant and develop than unfragmented counterparts. Overall, there is an established link between the surmised embryo quality score (combined cell number and morphology grade) and the pregnancy outcome. Studies have shown that patients who have embryos regarded as 'top quality' (over 7 blastomeres, less than 20 per cent fragmentation, day 3) have a good prognosis for achieving a pregnancy; however there is a high probability of multiple implantation if two embryos are transferred.[1] Multiple pregnancies carry a higher risk of miscarriage, maternal complications and premature delivery, therefore when multiple good-quality embryos are available to select from; the pressure to identify the single most viable embryo for transfer is increased. Extending the culture period until day 5 is one way to facilitate the selection process.

On day 5 of development the embryo will have many cells, which will have compacted and merged to form two distinct cell populations, separated by an expanded fluid filled cavity; the embryo is now a blastocyst. Blastocysts are also graded and this necessitates scoring the embryo according to the degree of expansion (i.e. looking to see how big it is and for the presence of a cavity and the thinning of the outer protective zona 'shell'), the integrity of cells of the inner part of the blastocyst (inner cell mass -ICM) and the outer cells forming the trophectoderm (TE). An alpha-numerical score is assigned to distinguish good-quality blastocysts; identified by a high number of cells in the ICM and tight knit cells of the TE.[2]

Assessments may be carried out at discreet time points throughout development (day 1–6) to build up a sequence of pictures, alternatively in recent years attention has moved to the use of time-lapse imaging systems. Time-lapse imaging permits numerous observations to be made, with images typically being acquired every 10–20 minutes. While the virtues of such analyses are widely extolled, randomised controlled trials demonstrating the efficacy of such an approach are still currently lacking.[3]

Studies comparing pregnancy rates following transfer of blastocyst or cleavage stage embryos have in the past produced conflicting results. However, the latest studies have generally concluded that for selected 'good prognosis' patients blastocyst transfer offers a significant advantage. Furthermore, when chromosome analysis was performed it was demonstrated that while 63 per cent of 8 cell embryos were abnormal only 48 per cent of the cells in the blastocyst were abnormal.[4] Taken together, it may be argued that extended culture to the blastocyst allows selection of the best-quality embryo for transfer and could reduce the likelihood of freezing non-viable embryos. Despite this, safety concerns over blastocyst culture linger and it has been suggested that prolonged laboratory culture could impact on early embryo development and on the long-term health of the child, thus continuing follow up studies of children conceived by IVF remains paramount, and decisions to transfer one or two embryos, and on which day of development, need to be carefully considered. It is important to discuss with your clinic the merits of each strategy based on your individual prognosis and the observed development of your cohort of embryos.

The quality of the embryo selected for transfer is obviously a key factor influencing the success of IVF. The importance of maternal and paternal lifestyle factors in relation to embryo quality are relatively unknown and it is possible that subtle differences in lifestyle factors during gametogenesis (development and maturation of eggs and sperm) could translate into differences in resultant embryo quality and chances of a live birth. Factors influencing egg and sperm development will be considered in turn in the next section.

3. Age

Embryo quality is a function of both egg and sperm quality, both of which decrease with advancing age. For women in particular, fertility is known to decline with age, as ovarian aging results in fewer eggs of lower quality. It is generally accepted that a woman is born with all the eggs that she will ever have and with advancing age this store (ovarian reserve) is gradually depleted. The progressive loss of eggs being most evident after the age of thirty-five, furthermore the quality of these eggs declines and the prevalence of chromosome abnormalities increases. Fertility is decreased by about half among women in their late thirties compared with women in their early twenties.[5]

Age-related decline in fertility is not as pronounced in men and the testes are able to continue producing sperm throughout adulthood. Detectable declines in semen parameters are evident post-thirty-five years, but male fertility doesn't appear to be affected before the age of fifty.[6] The decline in quality of the sperm with advancing age may be explained by the higher reported incidence of chromosome abnormalities and DNA damage in the sperm of older men.

The consensus is that chromosome abnormalities in embryos are more frequently associated with advanced patient age and declining IVF success rates. However, discernible differences in visual embryo quality may not always be evident, particularly at the earlier stages of development. It is theorised that in both sexes an age-dependent accumulation of damage due to several possible mechanisms, including for instance, a gradual increase in oxidative stress, which compromises the production of egg and sperm cells. Oxidative stress is something that occurs when reactive oxygen species (ROS), which are produced during normal cellular processes, are not counterbalanced by our antioxidant defences. In addition, this oxidative stress may be exacerbated by dietary and lifestyle factors, considered in the next section.

4. Body weight

Numerous reports highlight the importance of attaining an ideal weight prior to attempting to conceive. Body mass index (BMI), which is the ratio of body weight in kilograms (kg) to height in metres squared (m^2), is the most widely used assessment criterion used to gauge normality for a person's weight. A BMI of less than $18.5 kg/m^2$ is defined as underweight, 18.5–24.9 normal weight, 25–29.9 overweight and over $30 kg/m^2$ obese according to the WHO (World Health Organisation) classification. BMI calculations are not without shortcomings, as the measure does not account for lean body mass, nor does it provide any indication of the distribution of body fat; however, it is a standardised and easily reproduced measurement. Treatment with IVF is believed to be more effective in women who have a BMI between 19 and $30 kg/m^2$ and you may find that many IVF Clinics will have patient acceptance criteria, based around this range.

The reason BMI is given such attention is that, in order for the reproductive-endocrine (hormone) system to function correctly, women in particular require a minimum amount of body fat (adipose tissue) and available energy balance to meet their nutritional needs. The link between the hypothalamus in the brain; which regulates the pituitary gland and the release of sex hormones and body weight and composition has been well established. Studies of seasonal patterns of fertility, low birth rates during times of famine (Dutch *Hongerwinter*) and the prevalence of amenorrhoea (absent periods) in female athletes and women with eating disorders, all serve to illustrate how being underweight can alter sex hormone gonadotrophin concentrations through the release of gonadotrophin releasing hormone (GnRH). In underweight individuals it is plausible that this is due to decreased signalling of the hormone leptin, produced from adipose tissue to the hypothalamus.

At the other end of the spectrum, obesity impacts on the female reproductive system in a number of ways and is a well-documented cause of female subfertility. Obese women are less likely to get pregnant, are at increased risk of miscarriage and still birth, and are more likely to encounter health problems during pregnancy.[7] Moreover, rates of birth defects are increased with maternal obesity.

In obese women, metabolic disturbances of the hypothalamic-pituitary ovarian axis may be caused by excessive steroid (oestrogen) production from adipose tissue and by the elevated levels of the hormones; insulin and leptin. Oestrogen then suppresses the hypothalamic-pituitary axis, reducing the availability of GnRH, which at the pituitary stimulates the synthesis and secretion of the gonadotrophins; follicle-stimulating hormone (FSH) and luteinising hormone (LH). The disorderly activity of these two hormones impairs egg development and ovulation, leading to menstrual irregularities in up to 47 per cent of obese women.[8]

Infertility in couples trying to conceive naturally is almost three times higher among obese women; however the impact that raised BMI has on the outcome of IVF is not as clear. Over twenty-four studies, including more than 78,000 cycles have thus far reviewed the evidence of association between IVF success rates and female BMI. Of these, fourteen studies have reported no association with clinical pregnancy rates, although the combined analysis of these studies has been used to demonstrate lower live birth rates with increasing BMI by several investigators.

It is generally accepted that obese women require a longer duration and dose of ovarian stimulation (fertility drugs) and that they produce fewer eggs for collection; approximately 7–25 per cent lower yields for women with a BMI greater than $25kg/m^2$,[9] although evidence for differences in fertilisation or embryo development is less convincing. Three studies have reported lower fertilisation rates, while five refuted any association with BMI, and embryo score was found to be lower for women with a BMI of under $25kg/m^2$ in two of five studies. It is also not clear from the literature if embryo quality in successive cycles of fertility treatment is similar for the same couple and therefore it is difficult to say with any degree of certainty if weight loss would lead to improvements in embryo quality. Furthermore, inconsistent embryo-quality grading systems have prevented such analyses.

There is a general agreement that a mother's nutrition during the time before pregnancy to early pregnancy has an appreciable impact on live birth outcome: birth weights are significantly higher for babies born to overweight/ obese women compared to those of normal-weight women. This is not surprising, as maternal supply of nutrients is known to affect the growth and the development of the embryo/foetus, which will adapt its metabolism in order to thrive. However, such early adaptations are a source of serious concern, as size at birth is proposed to be related to the risk of developing diabetes and heart disease later in life.[10]

Potentially more concerning still, is the emerging data which indicates that these adaptations actually begin prior to conception and during egg development, leaving a lasting effect on the growth and development of the child. Metabolic adaptations have been observed in embryos derived from overweight and obese women, that may be inconsistent with further development and likelihood of pregnancy.[11]

This section has largely focused on female BMI, but increasing numbers of studies are emerging which suggest that male BMI is also an important consideration. As with women, endocrine changes associated with a BMI outside of the normal range can disrupt reproductive function. Hormone production may be compromised in men who are more than 20 per cent below their recommended weight. Additionally, hormone changes associated with obesity can result in reduced levels of testosterone and increased levels of oestrogen, subsequently affecting sperm production. This altered ratio could lead to decreased testis size, and damage to the sperm DNA.

Male obesity has been associated with increased time to conception, reduced pregnancy rates and a higher incidence of miscarriage. Obese men are more likely to exhibit a reduction in sperm quality, compared with those of normal weight. However, the relationship between BMI and independent assessment parameters of semen quality including ejaculate volume, sperm concentration and motility is more controversial; thirteen studies reporting no individual relationships and nine reporting negative associations with increasing BMI.[12] Lower numbers of normal motile sperm, may contribute to lower fertilisation rates and impaired sperm binding as reported for obese men and in animal models comparing obese and control subjects.[13] It has also previously been reported that rates of blastocyst formation are lower for embryos derived from obese males, with lower sperm counts, treated with ICSI.[14]

As has been reported for female obesity, male obesity is also reported to increase the susceptibility of the offspring to developing health problems later in life. Recent evidence from animal models supports the assertion that male BMI has trans-generational effects,[15] i.e. molecular changes from impaired sperm production as a consequence of obesity are transmitted to the embryo and consequently affect the development and health of the child.

5. Diet/nutrition

As we have seen in Chapter 4, a poor diet may result in deficiencies in key vitamins, minerals and trace elements required for reproductive processes including maintenance of normal cellular function and hormone production. Restriction diets, excluding certain food groups, or an extreme calorie deficit will deprive the body of vital nutrients required for energy, cell division, biosynthesis and repair. Similarly, caloric excess and intake of energy-dense foods, high in fats and refined sugars and low in other vital nutrients, can have direct and indirect negative effects on reproductive function. This section will focus on the specific impact of exposing the developing eggs and sperm to differing nutrients and oxidative stress.

Good dietary practices will ensure that the body receives an adequate balance of macronutrients (protein, fats and carbohydrates) and micronutrients (vitamins and minerals). Men and women need 60–70g of protein a day (20 per cent of diet). A protein deficiency and deficiencies in specific amino acids can lead to compromised egg, sperm and embryo development; studies have shown that the specific utilisation of individual amino acids is linked to embryo viability.[16] Dietary fatty acids include saturated, monounsaturated and polyunsaturated fatty acid and are required for hormone balance. Essential, unsaturated fatty acids should make up 20–25 per cent of diet. Diets high in saturated fatty acid, raised omega-6 and trans fats, and low omega-3 fat ratios can compromise reproductive function, including egg and embryo development. Raised triglyceride and free fatty acid levels in the follicular fluid (fluid bathing the eggs in the ovary) can promote fat accumulation and impaired egg development. Furthermore, embryos arresting at the cleavage stages of development have been shown to contain significantly more triglyceride than those capable of forming blastocysts.[17] Studies have also shown that a diet high in omega-6 polyunsaturated fatty acids may affect ovulation and the incorporation of omega-3 fatty acids can enhance ovulation.[18] The significant effects of fatty acids on male fertility have also been well documented in animal and human studies; several studies have reported lower blood and semen concentrations of omega-3 fatty acids for infertile men compared to fertile counterparts. Carbohydrates account for 50 per cent of diet and are required for balanced hormone and blood sugar levels. Carbohydrates should be complex, derived from slow-release whole foods (whole grains, fruit and vegetables) rather than processed foods and refined simple carbohydrates. Evidence from animal and human studies indicate that eggs exposed to high glucose concentrations display signs of compromised development and metabolism.

Deficiencies in certain micro-nutrients (vitamins and minerals) and phytochemicals, have been linked to miscarriage and hormone imbalances. Vitamins and minerals are powerful antioxidants and can be attained from dietary and natural sources including; fruit, vegetables, herbs and spices. Specific pre-conception supplements are also available and several clinical trials have examined the efficacy of pre-treatment (usually minimum of three months) supplementation to reduce oxidative stress. Reactive oxygen species (ROS) are a by-product of reduction-oxidation reactions and play an important role in numerous physiological reproductive processes. In healthy individuals reactive oxygen species and antioxidants (natural enzymatic and/or dietary) remain in balance; however, an imbalance will result in oxidative stress and can lead to cellular damage and poor-quality eggs. Similarly high levels of ROS in semen have been associated with sperm DNA damage and dysfunction. Poor-quality eggs and sperm will invariably result in lower fertilisation rates and poorer embryo quality. There has been inconclusive debate about the efficacy of pre-conception antioxidant supplements; generally studies have supported their use for select cases of infertility.

6. Exercise

The evidence appraising the effects of exercise on egg and sperm quality is often contradictory, thus definitive guidelines on the optimum amount/ and type of exercise for optimum fertility are lacking, furthermore the effects vary from one individual to another. By and large, moderate exercise is reported to improve reproductive outcomes in both men and women. The physiological benefits of exercise include improved metabolism and circulation which stimulates the endocrine glands, which secrete sex hormones. Exercise reduces oxidative stress by increasing cellular antioxidant defences, but vigorous exercise generally reduces success, in all but those classified as obese.[19]

The available evidence would suggest that women who exercise for approximately 30 minutes a day suffer fewer ovulatory disorders. However, more than an hour of vigorous exercise a day can lead to a decrease in the production of sex hormones and cause periods to stop. Ovulation is often impaired if body fat is less than 12 per cent or more than 30 percent.

In men regular exercise decreases fat and increases lean muscle, leading to less oestrogen and more testosterone and thus improved sperm production. As reported for women the type and intensity of exercise is worthy of consideration, especially as the question of an association between cycling and infertility has been a source of much debate. The theoretical premise is that hard, narrow bicycle seats can put pressure on the perineum, reducing the blood flow to the genitals – recent studies, however, suggest that modern saddles spread the pressure out laterally, mitigating the risks. Nevertheless, tight clothing such as cycling shorts or running tights worn during exercise may increase heat around the testicles, and scrotal heating due to clothing or hot tub and sauna use may affect testicular function and are best avoided, as are testosterone supplements or prohormones to gain muscle.

It is thus generally advisable that normal-weight

individuals should exercise at the 'public health' rate of 150 minutes weekly; i.e. 30 minutes of moderate-intensity activity five days a week.

7. Alcohol, caffeine, smoking and stress

Public health information states that if a couple are attempting to conceive and either partner regularly drink more than 1 unit of alcohol a day this will lessen their chance of success with IVF.[20] An increased risk of IVF failure has been reported for women consuming at least 4 drinks a week in the month prior to treatment.[21] In men, acetaldehyde (a breakdown product of alcohol metabolism) has been linked to abnormalities in developing sperm. Abstinence from alcohol is thus recommended prior and during treatment and pregnancy.

A limited number of studies have considered the impact of caffeine consumption on reproductive outcomes, and no references are available to ascertain the impact on embryo development. Moderate to high caffeine consumption is reported to increase time to conception by up to 50 per cent.[22] Caffeine is both a diuretic and a stimulant, and moderate to high consumption can deplete the body of water and minerals and stimulate the production of the stress hormone cortisol. In women caffeine consumption increases the risk of miscarriage and in men there is some evidence linking high caffeine intake prior to conception and increased risk of premature birth.

Smoking is a modifiable factor known to influence

IVF success, reducing pregnancy rates by as much as half in some reports and increasing the risk of miscarriage. Smoking compromises egg quality and ovarian response and also impacts on the likelihood of implantation, as demonstrated in a donor egg (non-smoker) to recipient (heavy smoker) study.[23] Passive smoking also poses a risk, as cotinine; a nicotine metabolite, has been isolated from the follicular fluid of the ovaries of non-smokers and found to be associated with an increased risk of embryo implantation failure, compared to results from women without traces of the compound in their fluid.[24] Furthermore, some studies have reported that men who smoke are more likely to have reduced sperm counts, motility, morphology and reduced testosterone levels. Other researchers have found no significant differences between smokers and non-smokers in terms of traditional semen parameters, but reported significantly higher levels of sperm DNA fragmentation in the sperm of smokers. Broadly speaking, smoking results in fewer eggs, poorer sperm quality, lower fertilisation rates and thus fewer embryos available for selection for transfer or cryopreservation, but it is also conceivable that, as smoking reduces cell replication in organs, the embryo development/ cell division may also be compromised.

Stress can also influence reproductive outcomes; stress hormones (adrenaline and cortisol) disrupt the hypothalamic pituitary axis and the secretion of gonadotrophins compromising egg and sperm quality. Anecdotally, it is reported that exercise, massage, breathing techniques, and the establishment of positive sleeping habits may all help to reduce stress hormone levels.

8. Strategies for improving ovarian response to IVF stimulation (egg quality and quantity)

In assisted conception (IVF), egg quality plays a critical role in treatment success. Ovarian reserve (likely number of eggs) can be ascertained from blood tests and ultrasound scans of the ovaries, but these fail to correlate with quality. An egg's quality is a measure of its developmental capability, which is progressively acquired during its growth within its follicle (egg sac) in the ovary and is best described by the capacity of the egg to sustain early embryo development. An egg's growth and development is dependent on the energy / nutrient supply it acquires from the bathing in the follicular fluid and its internal reserves. As previously stated, there are well established differences in the follicular environment of eggs from obese and normal weight women and suggested differences in the fat reserves contained within the eggs, which can compromise embryo quality through impaired energy production and sensitivity to oxidative stress. Strategies to combat oxidative stress may thus improve egg and embryo quality.

It is clear that the obese environment is detrimental to embryo development, although the exact mechanisms underlying this are only just beginning to emerge. Several studies have shown that moderate weight loss may improve reproductive outcomes. One study estimated a 4 per cent increased likelihood of pregnancy for every unit decrease in BMI until a BMI of less than $30kg/m^2$ is achieved.[25] It is widely believed that hormone signalling may be corrected once a healthy weight is attained, with modest weight loss shown to induce ovulation in 50 per cent of previously anovulatory overweight women.[26] While changes in BMI impact likelihood of conceiving naturally, for those with specific causes of infertility requiring IVF, the outcomes from repeat IVF treatment cycles are unlikely to vary significantly, once other confounding factors have been accounted for. For example, a 3.1kg weight loss has been shown to improve egg quality, but this was unrelated to pregnancy rates.[27] Possibly owing to the fact that weight loss is a long term commitment and any improvements to egg quality as a consequence of decreasing BMI may be offset by the known detrimental effects that advancing maternal age has on egg quality.

A further point for consideration is that in many of the studies weight loss is assumed to be as a consequence of altered food consumption, but nothing is known about how the balance of consumption of macronutrients, such as carbohydrate and protein differed between cycles. Without performing dietary assessments, it is not possible to ascertain the influence of dietary change on treatment outcome. Calorie restriction (crash dieting) may result in rapid weight reduction, however women who lose weight very rapidly to meet a target BMI are also at risk of rapidly regaining the weight lost and 60–86 per cent of weight lost is regained after three years. Extreme dieting could also have serious future consequences, as demonstrated in reports of increased incidences of foetal abnormalities in women who achieve a pregnancy after bariatric surgery.

Weight reduction is best achieved with a combination of dietary advice, exercise and physiological support. Advice to quit smoking is best sought well in advance of attempting conception and it is prudent to consider abstaining from alcohol, limiting caffeine intake and eating a nutritionally balanced diet. The benefits of taking any pre-conception food supplements will need to be considered in the context of your individual lifestyle factors/ exposures, as each person's nutritional needs will vary according to the stresses to which they are exposed; in any case food supplements should only be used according to recommended doses. Too high an intake of one particular vitamin or mineral may result in a depletion in the levels of another – for example a high intake of zinc can reduce the uptake of iron and vice versa. Similarly, vitamins E and C are known to act synergistically. All women attempting to conceive are advised to take folate and B vitamins according to Department of Health guidelines (generally 400mcg/ daily) and to include folate rich foods in their diet to reduce the risk of neural tube defects.

Dehydroepiandrosterone (DHEA), a supplement unlicensed in Europe but available online has been reported to improve egg quality. The potential side effects and long-term actions have not been addressed and evidence does not support the routine use of DHEA as an 'add-on' in IVF cycles. Similarly convincing evidence is unavailable to support follicular priming with oestrogen or the combined oral contraceptive pill. Evidence supporting adjunct therapies to optimise ovarian responsiveness and subsequent egg quality and embryo quality is by and large lacking, the possible exception being metformin, which may be beneficial for women with polycystic ovaries, reducing the risk of ovarian hyperstimulation.

The importance of adopting evidence based, healthy preconception lifestyle habits, particularly attaining a healthy weight before pregnancy must not be underplayed, as studies have shown that the negative effects of poor maternal health preconception can extend beyond poor conception rates and may influence the future health of the child.

9. Strategies for improving semen parameters

Oxidative stress has been linked to DNA fragmentation, and antioxidant therapy (food supplements) is one proposed solution to improve sperm quality and thus improve embryo quality and the probability of successful implantation. DNA damage is reported to be reduced in men taking oral doses of vitamins C and E. However, no current treatments offer clear, proven benefits.

Obesity is linked with chronic systemic inflammation and generation of reactive oxygen species (ROS), together with higher levels of sperm oxidative stress and increased testicular temperature due to excess scrotal adipose tissue. Overcoming obesity, through gradual weight loss as a result of improvements in diet and exercise is reported to improve circulating levels of hormones, including serum testosterone levels. Aromatase inhibitors can also be used to pharmacologically restore normal hormone levels and potentially improve semen parameters in obese men – whether this will lead to improved fertilisation rates and embryo development remains to be investigated. Obesity is, however, often linked to other health complaints, and drugs prescribed for treating conditions such as diabetes and hypertension may affect sperm production.

Exposure to environmental pollutants, such as bisphenol A (BPA) used in plastic containers, has been correlated with increased rates of miscarriage and poorer sperm quality. Exposure to environmental oestrogens, pesticides and herbicides may be reduced by choosing organic foods, drinking filtered water and rinsing fruit and vegetables.

The virtues of a Mediterranean diet, high in essential fatty acids, have been well-regarded by many, based on an association between high dietary intake of omega-3, and low saturated-fat intake and reduced odds of poor sperm motility. Sperm membranes contain a high concentration of omega-3 fatty acids; these polyunsaturated fatty acids are chemically unstable and therefore highly sensitive to oxidative stress. Carnitines (an amino acid derivative) facilitate fatty acid oxidation and protect cell membranes from ROS-induced damage and studies have also shown oral supplementation with carnitine can improve sperm motility. Similarly selenium may protect against oxidative damage and adequate zinc intake is needed for normal sperm motility. It is, however, important to note that excessive intake can have adverse pro-oxidant effects and the effects of supplementation will depend on pre-treatment semen characteristics and individual oxidative stress levels.

10. Conclusion

There is gathering evidence to suggest that the maternal environment prior to conception impacts on egg quality, maturation and post-fertilisation embryo competence. In addition, sperm produced under conditions of oxidative stress may have lower fertilising capability and post-fertilisation this could also result in reduced embryo health, leading to increased rates of miscarriage.

Embryo competence can be determined using assessments of cell morphology and time recordings of development or by chromosome screening techniques, however the ultimate test is the ability of the embryo to implant and give rise to a healthy baby. Embryo grading is not an exact science and there are a multitude of factors which interlink to influence embryo development and the likelihood of pregnancy. None the less, the incremental gains that can be achieved by making marginal lifestyle adjustments to optimise egg and sperm development should not be discounted. The key message is that diet and exercise should be well balanced and moderation in all lifestyle factors is fundamental.

References

1. Gerris, J., et al., 1999. 'Prevention of twin pregnancy after in-vitro fertilization or intracytoplasmic sperm injection based on strict embryo criteria: a prospective randomized clinical trial'. *Human reproduction* 14(10), pp.2581–2587; https://doi.org/10.1093/humrep/14.10.2581.

2. Gardner, D. and Schoolcraft, W., 1999. 'In vitro culture of human blastocysts', *Towards reproductive certainty:the Plenary Proceedings of the 11th World Congress* (1999) pp. 378-388.

3. Bolton, V., Leary, C. et al., 2015, 'How should we choose the "best" embryo? A commentary on behalf of the BFS and the ACE', *Human fertility*, 18 (3) pp. 156–164.

4. Magli, M. C., Gianaroli, L. and Ferraretti, A. P., 2001, 'Chromosomal abnormalities in embryos', *Molecular and cellular endocrinology*, 183 Supplement 1, pp. S29–S34.

5. ASRM, 2013, 'Criteria for number of embryos to transfer: a committee opinion', *Fertility and sterility*, 99 (1), pp. 44–6.

6. Ibid.

7. Balen, A. H., and Anderson, R. A., 2007. 'Impact of obesity on female reproductive health': British Fertility Society, Policy and Practice Guidelines, *Human Fertility*, 10(4), pp. 195–206.

8. ARSM, 2008, 'Obesity and reproduction: an educational bulletin', *Fertility and sterility*, 90(5 Supplement), pp. S21–S29.

9. Ibid.

10. Barker, D. J., 1990, 'The fetal and infant origins of adult disease', *BMJ (Clinical research ed.)*, 301(6761), p. 1111.

11. Leary, C., Leese, H. J., and Sturmey, R. G., 2015, 'Human embryos

from overweight and obese women display phenotypic and metabolic abnormalities', *Human reproduction*, 30(1), pp. 122–32.

12. Davidson, L. M., et al., 2015, 'Deleterious effects of obesity upon the hormonal and molecular mechanisms controlling spermatogenesis and male fertility', *Human fertility*, 7273(April), pp. 1–10.

13. Palmer, N. O. et al., 2012, 'Impact of obesity on male fertility, sperm function and molecular composition', *Spermatogenesis*, 2(4), pp. 253–263.

14. Schliep, K. C. et al., 2015, 'Effect of male and female body mass index on pregnancy and live birth success after in vitro fertilization', *Fertility and sterility*, 103(2), pp. 388–395.

15. Palmer, 2012, op. cit.

16. Leary, et al., 2015, op. cit.

17. Ibid.

18. Mehendale, S. S. et al., 2009, 'Oxidative stress-mediated essential polyunsaturated fatty acid alterations in female infertility', *Human fertility*, 12(1), pp. 28–33.

19. Wise, L. A., et al., 2012, 'A prospective cohort study of physical activity and time to pregnancy', *Fertility and sterility*, 97(5), pp. 1136–1142.e1–4.

20. NICE, Fertility Guidance and guidelines.

21. Nicolau, P. et al., 2014. 'Alcohol consumption and in vitro fertilization: a review of the literature',*Gynecological endocrinology : the official journal of the International Society of Gynecological Endocrinology*, 30(11), pp. 759–763.

22. Hassan, M. A., and Killick, S. R., 2004, 'Negative lifestyle is associated with a significant reduction in fecundity', *Fertility and Sterility*, 81(2), pp. 384–392.

23. Soares, S. R., et al., 2007, 'Cigarette smoking affects uterine receptiveness', *Human reproduction*, 22(2), pp. 543–547.24.

24. Benedict, M. D., et al., 2011, 'Cotinine concentrations in follicular fluid as a measure of second-hand tobacco smoke exposure in women

undergoing in vitro fertilization: inter-matrix comparisons with urine and temporal variability', *Chemosphere*, 84(1), pp.110–6.'

25. van der Steeg, J. W. et al., 2008. Obesity affects spontaneous pregnancy chances in subfertile, ovulatory women. *Human reproduction (Oxford, England)*, 23(2), pp.324–8.

26. ARSM, 2008, op. cit.

27. Ibid.

CHAPTER 6

Egg Freezing — the Answer to Female Fertility Preservation?

Tracey Sainsbury, Lead Fertility Counsellor
at the London Women's Clinic

1. Introduction

In this chapter I'd like to provide an overview of the past, present and also a glimpse into the future of egg freezing and fertility preservation.

As a specialist fertility counsellor associated with several leading London fertility clinics, I have worked with women who have chosen not to pursue egg freezing, women who have chosen to and who happily have one or two eggs frozen, women with twenty-plus eggs frozen, and also women who feel concerned with 'only' thirty-plus eggs frozen.

If you are considering freezing your eggs, I hope this chapter will empower you to make an informed choice. I also hope to outline the benefits of counselling prior to and during the egg-freezing process.

To begin, a few interesting facts about eggs:

- A female foetus begins to produce eggs from 9 weeks' gestation, reaching an optimum at around 20 weeks' gestation of 5–7 million eggs. You may find it fascinating to know that the egg that created you was developed as your mother was growing inside her mother's uterus.

- Egg quantity begins to decline at around 20 weeks gestation; unlike men who continually produce sperm, women will be born with 1–2 million immature eggs remaining. This decline in the number of eggs is called ovarian follicle atresia and is the process where immature eggs inside immature follicles degenerate and are reabsorbed. Research from two Scottish universities revealed that by the time a woman reaches thirty she would routinely have lost around 90 per cent of her egg reserve.[1]

- During each menstrual cycle around 20 ovarian follicles begin to develop – these are called antral follicles – routinely, one continues to develop to maturity and the egg grows attached to the inner wall of the follicle. As it reaches maturity it detaches in anticipation of being released through ovulation. As only one follicle becomes dominant each month, only one egg is routinely released, with a woman ovulating around 400 times in her lifetime.

2. A brief history of egg freezing

Egg freezing (or human oocyte cryopreservation) is only a few years younger than in vitro fertilisation (IVF), which was successful for the first time in 1978.

The first successful pregnancy from thawed previously frozen eggs was reported in Australia in 1986.[2]

As access to IVF increased, so did the desire of some women to freeze their eggs, initially attempted only as a way to preserve fertility for single cancer sufferers or women experiencing other medical conditions that had or could have a detrimental impact on their fertility. Over time the number of women wishing to freeze their eggs for religious, social and ethical reasons has increased,[3] in preference to creating embryos to be frozen following a fertility treatment cycle, where the ovaries were stimulated producing a surplus of eggs.

3. Vitrification process

Early trials used a slow-freezing method, and though eggs froze, the success rates for achieving a pregnancy after surviving the thawing process remained low even where many eggs had been frozen.

In order to understand the difference between slow freezing and the more commonly used vitrification process (a cryopreservation technique that leads to a glass-like solidification), it can help to think about chickens! Frozen chickens to be precise (apologies to any vegetarians reading this). If you take a frozen chicken from the freezer and place on the countertop to thaw, you will see a white ice crust form as it begins to thaw. The same occurs when we thaw eggs. Although human eggs are the largest cells in the female body, they are also very fragile. So, as ice crystals form and expand in size, their sharp edges cause damage to the eggshell, preventing it from being a stable enough structure for fertilisation to take place.

Vitrification is a much faster way of freezing eggs; the process includes dehydrating the eggs, removing the water that can cause ice-crystal formation during thawing, and adding a cryopreservant that acts as a sort of anti-freeze.

Rather than actually freezing the eggs, the vitrification process turns the egg's outer shell into a glass-like state, preventing damage during flash freezing to the genetic material inside. Eggs stored can be left in that state until ready to warm, rather than thaw.

Research studies comparing the success rates between slow freezing and vitrification methods of storing eggs bring vitrification out on top, most citing 80 per cent plus thaw/warm success rates when vitrification is used.[4] Hence, vitrification is most often the favoured choice by clinics in the UK today when storing eggs to preserve fertility.

4. Current UK laws on egg freezing

It is now several years since egg freezing and using frozen eggs, especially in egg-donation treatment, became more commonplace in the UK, and in 2013 egg freezing was deemed to be no longer an experimental practice.[5]

The current UK laws allow women to freeze eggs routinely for up to ten years. Once fertilised, the resulting embryos can be stored for a further ten years, but storage can be extended in some circumstances. For example, if a woman has or is likely to develop a condition which can impact detrimentally on her fertility, then the law gives permission for storage to be extended up to a maximum of fifty-five years. In order to extend the storage period a clinician has to confirm in writing that there is a likelihood of premature infertility.

Conditions where fertility may be detrimentally impacted upon include:

- Premature ovarian failure or a family history of premature menopause
- Recurrent ovarian cysts
- Severe endometriosis

5. Most common reasons why women choose to freeze their eggs

Some women choose to freeze their eggs due to fertility issues (such as those mentioned above). Others choose to freeze their eggs due to busy careers delaying motherhood. Indeed, in these modern times when companies such as Facebook and Apple are offering egg-freezing treatment free of charge to employees as part of their healthcare package, this appears to be a growing trend. Another reason for egg freezing is simply that women feel that they have not yet found their life partner with whom they would like to have a family. In fact, the European Society of Human Reproduction and Embryology Task Force on Ethics and Law investigated the rise of egg freezing and found that the most common reason for egg freezing was that women had not yet found their ideal partner with whom to have a family.[6]

6. Egg freezing – choosing a clinic

There are many factors to consider when choosing a fertility clinic, but when thinking of egg freezing it is important to select a clinic that is experienced in both freezing eggs and using frozen eggs within IVF treatment cycles.

Some clinics have egg banks attached that may recruit egg donors and freeze eggs for use by recipients; some may have busy oncology centres associated with them and have experience in freezing eggs prior to chemotherapy. Others perhaps have experience of importing frozen eggs donated from overseas for treatment in the UK. It is important to ask clinics about their thawing/rewarming processes in addition to asking how many egg-freezing cycles they do each year.

A great source for clinic listings is the Human Fertilisation and Embryology Authority website: www. hfea.gov.uk. Once you have made your shortlist of clinics,

I would advise visiting them in person to pick up an information pack. If the clinic you are considering offers an information evening or open day, I would suggest going along. Being comfortable will not necessarily impact on your success rate but can make the process much less stressful if you like the clinic where you will be attending your appointments.

Some clinics offer a package for women wanting to have an overview of their fertility, a sort of Fertility MOT, for anyone wanting to be a 'Mother Of Tomorrow'. If you are comparing clinics by price, make sure you're aware of what is included and what is added on as an extra.

An initial consultation can appear to be excellent value, but if you pay more for an internal pelvic ultrasound scan, an additional payment for a blood test or tests, and there is a further cost for a follow-up appointment to receive the results and plan treatment, it can be more cost-effective to find a package deal, especially if you are just fact-finding and exploring options.

When comparing clinics do remember that the success rates published only represent the results of the women who have had treatment at that clinic. It's also important to ensure results shared relate to women freezing eggs for their own use. Women donating eggs for the treatment of others are selected, based on their age, medical history, their wider families' medical history and, primarily, their fertility. So, although experience of using frozen eggs is beneficial, the success rates with donated eggs will routinely be much higher than average.

7. Initial consultation, hormone testing and preparation for egg collection

If your initial consultation is part of a comprehensive fertility assessment, it will most often include a blood test, an internal pelvic ultrasound scan and a consultation with the fertility specialist as a minimum. If your initial consultation does not include tests, it will be an opportunity for you to explore your hopes and expectations and for the specialist to review your medical history and provide a framework of tests to undertake prior to a treatment plan being put in place.

The blood test most used when considering egg freezing is the anti-Müllerian hormone blood test referred to as AMH. This test measures the anti-Müllerian hormone level present in your blood. It is a test that can be performed on any day of your monthly cycle and most clinics state that the results are valid for around a year.

The AMH blood test is sometimes referred to as the 'ovarian reserve' test. Your AMH level is used in conjunction with the findings from your internal pelvic ultrasound scan to provide the specialist with an overview of your fertility, which enables them to estimate how likely you are to respond to medication used to stimulate your ovaries.

If you have a high AMH level it may suggest to the specialist that there is a possibility of you over-responding to medication to stimulate your ovaries. If it is very high, it can suggest that you have polycystic ovaries. If it is an unexpectedly low result, it can suggest that egg quality may be impacted in addition to the number of eggs that may be collected if your ovaries are stimulated. A low AMH can also reassure a fertility specialist that you can tolerate a higher dose of medication to stimulate your ovaries with less of a risk of your ovaries over-responding.

Some laboratories use different scales when performing tests, so checking the internet to see what your results mean isn't advised as you don't know which scale will be used by the clinic.

The internal pelvic ultrasound scan provides lots of information; it may be performed by the specialist, an ultra-sonographer or a specialist nurse who has had additional training in fertility scanning. They will be looking at the results to check your uterine cavity. Having awareness of the day you are on of your monthly cycle enables the specialist to check that the endometrium, the uterus lining, looks as it should.

The scan will also check the uterine cavity for contraindications to pregnancy. If there's a sign of anything detrimental (a polyp or fibroid, for example) they will let you know so that when you are ready to try to conceive you can include having it checked or treated as part of your preparation for pregnancy plans.

The scan will also include looking at your ovaries to determine their health and how active they are. Depending on the day of your cycle they will be looking for antral follicles – these are 'resting' follicles that have the potential to develop, though routinely in our monthly cycle only one goes on to be the dominant follicle – and also to ensure there are no unexpected cysts or abnormalities.

Depending on the clinic and the results of your AMH and pelvic ultrasound scan, additional blood tests may be requested which include your follicle stimulating hormone (FSH) and luteinizing hormone (LH). These are both gonadotropins: hormones produced by the pituitary gland to stimulate the gonads. Within the ovaries, the FSH stimulates the growth of immature follicles and the LH helps to mature the egg with a surge of the hormone-triggering ovulation from the dominant follicle.

When you have your results, your specialist will be able to advise you of the approximate number of follicles that may be recruited as your ovaries are stimulated during a treatment cycle and go on to tell you an approximate number of eggs that may be collected that are suitable for freezing. The specialist will also explain that there are risks and implications, which include:

- Not responding to the medication and the cycle needing to be abandoned

- Over-responding to the medication, and if you develop over hyperstimulation syndrome (see page 185) then hospital treatment may be required

- There being no eggs collected

- There being no mature eggs collected

- Eggs collected and frozen may not survive when thawed/warmed

- Eggs surviving being thawed/warmed then not fertilising

- Embryos created from previously frozen eggs not continuing to develop

- Multiple pregnancies (if two or more embryos created from previously frozen eggs are transferred)

- Eggs not being used if you conceive the family you hope for without needing to use the eggs or if you decide not to try to conceive

- Embryos created from previously frozen eggs not being required once your family is complete

If you decide to proceed with treatment or are considering it, the consultant may create a treatment plan for you. This will include the approximate days you will need to attend the clinic for internal scans to initially observe and then monitor the number of follicles developing on each ovary and the medication protocol and a prescription for your medication.

Your treatment medication plan will be designed for you around your test results and may be a long-protocol (or standard) cycle, a short- (or flare-) protocol and a mild (or micro-flare) cycle.

A long-protocol cycle includes medication to suppress the ovaries prior to stimulation; this enables the stimulatory medication to stimulate the ovaries without interference from the natural hormones produced during your menstrual cycle.

A short- or flare-protocol cycle will use medication to optimise the number of follicles that will develop alongside your naturally produced hormones. There is not a right or wrong protocol and medication is not a 'one size fits all' package. Your consultant will advise which protocol and medications will promote the best outcome for you based on your individual test results.

You can often purchase your medication at the clinic, but I always suggest that you do compare prices. Some pharmacies, including those in supermarkets and online, may sell private fertility drugs on a not-for-profit basis or at lower costs than the clinic.

You will also need the results of your rubella screening and a smear test result from within the last three years.

There are several consent forms that need to be signed in the clinic that confirm your consent to treatment to stimulate the ovaries, collect the eggs and freeze them on your behalf. In addition to providing consent to store the eggs for your use in the future, you will also be asked to confirm your wishes regarding your stored eggs in the unlikely event that should you die during the storage period or become mentally incapacitated. The consent forms are important: take time to read them and ensure you are comfortable with your decisions prior to handing them in to the clinic. If you have made plans for eggs to be used in the event of your death or mental incapacitation, it is important you let your loved ones know too.

The first year's storage fee is often included in the egg-freezing treatment cycle, you may have the option to pay a fixed fee for a certain number of years' storage or pay annually.

Your treatment will be costed for you; all clinics have to provide transparent pricing; you can find a list of clinics on the HFEA website and each will have a current price list available to download.

After meeting with a consultant, you may have some time with a nurse or specialist health-care assistant who will ensure you have retained the information shared within your appointment. There can be a lot to take in and if you're attending without a partner, it can be a good idea to have a friend with you. Do ask questions and find out who to contact if you have questions after leaving the clinic.

Some clinics book a routine counselling appointment prior to your treatment commencing, others offer it in line with the current regulations. But you can choose whether to attend or not.

8. Counselling

Fertility clinics in the UK are legally obliged to ensure that counselling is available for patients exploring any sort of fertility treatment. As discussed in Chapter 1 Counselling is important, especially in the case of donor assistance.

However, counselling is not mandatory or even routine for women hoping to freeze eggs, as clinics often assume it is not needed if patients aren't hoping to conceive at that time.

Counselling provides space to recognise and discuss the potential emotional impact that egg freezing can have. Post-egg freezing, women often feel a sense of elation – a sense that they have done something positive towards preserving their future fertility. For others, coming out of the egg-freezing process raises concerns about their future fertility (if the process has resulted in few or no eggs to be frozen, for example). Participating in counselling helps women to explore their feelings about the egg-freezing process and discuss their hopes and/or fears for their future fertility in a safe and confidential environment.

For women freezing eggs because of a medical condition such as cancer, it can bring a sense of relief that they are able to do something positive prior to beginning treatment for a condition that may impact their fertility.

9. To freeze or not to freeze

The initial consultation will have given you an idea of the potential number of eggs that may be collected if you were to proceed with a treatment cycle to stimulate your ovaries.

If freezing is an option that is offered to you, whether the results were positive, negative, encouraging or discouraging, it is up to you whether you decide to proceed or not. The specialist's job is not to tell you what to do, rather to provide sufficient information for you to make an informed decision.

Many clinics in the UK treat women with donated eggs up to the age of fifty and some up to fifty-four. The HFEA state on their website that treatment using donated eggs can offer success rates of around 25–40 per cent, higher than with conventional IVF. This can be an important factor if considering not freezing your own eggs and instead accessing donated eggs as an alternative.

Other good sources of support include:

- Gateway Women for single women who had hoped to or who assumed they would be a parent but for many different reasons currently aren't
- Fertility Friends and clinic support groups for those proceeding with treatment

10. The treatment cycle

Having made the decision to proceed you will have had all of your fertility and mandatory screening tests completed, you will have signed your consent forms, purchased your medication from the clinic or pharmacy and have a copy of your treatment schedule. You will have met with the nursing team to be taught how to administer your medication.

Calling the clinic on day 1 of your period will determine what medication to take when, and when to book in for your first scan.

Anxiety around the first few injections is normal; ensuring you have plenty of time can stop you feeling rushed. Some people prefer to have a friend or partner with them; others prefer to get on with it alone. There isn't a right or wrong way – whatever works best for you.

A scan is booked usually for day 3 of your period, confirming the number of antral follicles that can hopefully be developed by the stimulatory medication. If you are on a long protocol the scan also confirms that the suppression medication worked. Women are all unique, so it is impossible to confirm exactly how an individual will respond to the medication. Your next scan appointment will be booked and medication dosage confirmed.

The medication isn't hallucinogenic, but it can make you more aware of your emotions, so mood swings, tearfulness in addition to a bloating feeling are all usual. The bloating can increase as you become more physically aware of the increasing activity in your ovaries.

Your regular scans over the coming week can bring reassurance that you are responding well to the medication (around 10 per cent of women don't respond well). Your medication may be increased, reduced or changed depending on how you react. Your specialist will continue to work to optimise your personal treatment; slight changes to your treatment plan can be frustrating, and recognising it is not an exact plan from the beginning can help to alleviate some of the frustrations.

Occasionally, the specialist may recommend abandoning the cycle. If so, ensure you have all of the facts and that a follow-up appointment is booked to provide an opportunity for you to ask any questions and plan the next steps. Also, do ask if you can meet with a counsellor if you feel more support would be beneficial.

Occasionally your ovaries can respond too well to the stimulatory medication. Over hyperstimulation syndrome (OHSS) occurs when over-stimulated ovaries release chemicals into the bloodstream promoting a build-up of fluids in the abdomen and thorax. Your regular scans will alert a specialist to a heightened risk of OHSS, but if you experience any of the symptoms below it's important that you let the clinic know or seek medical help immediately:

- Swelling and bloating in the abdomen
- Severe pain in the lower abdomen
- Breathing difficulties
- Extreme thirst
- Reduced urination
- Feeling faint

Reassuringly, most cycles do progress with minimal problems, but it's important to be aware of the symptoms of OHSS so you can act accordingly if needed.

When your scan shows that your follicles have reached a point where they are ready to have the eggs inside matured (the lead follicles reaching a diameter of 18mm or more) your final trigger injection is given at a specific time, approximately thirty-six hours before your egg-collection procedure.

11. Egg-collection procedure

Egg-collection procedures are usually carried out in an operating theatre and you may be on a ward, in a cubicle or have a private room before and following your procedure.

Your egg-collection procedure is sometimes performed under a conscious sedation, rather than a general anaesthetic. A combination of medications is often used, including a sedative to help you relax and an anaesthetic to help block any pain.

You will now be familiar with the internal ultrasound-scanning probe, but may not be aware that they have an opening through the middle for a very fine retractable needle. While you are sedated, the specialist will guide the probe to align with the suitably large follicles and insert the needle through the vaginal wall to aspirate each of the follicles, draining off the fluid and within it the egg. The eggs are just about visible to the naked eye.

The length of time your egg collection procedure takes depends on the number of follicles produced, but on average is 20–30 minutes. After you have rested, eaten and hydrated you are allowed to go home; it is usual that a friend or relative is required to ensure you get home safely. You will not be able to drive for 24 hours after your procedure.

The fluid and eggs are taken to the lab by the

embryologists. Once there, the embryologist is able to count the eggs and confirm the number collected. Each egg is inspected and the cumulus, the cloud of cells surrounding each egg, is removed. The mature eggs can then be vitrified (frozen) and the number confirmed with you later the same day or early the following day.

You may then experience any number of feelings: pleased that you went through the process, feel the need to freeze more eggs, feel broody and experience a strong desire to become a parent now, feel sad that you aren't trying to conceive now, frustrated at the number of eggs collected and stored for you. If you're thinking about conceiving or having more treatment I always recommend not rushing, taking some time before booking a follow-up appointment. The hormones may take some time to leave your body and for you to get back to your former self.

However you may be feeling, counselling support is available to you via the clinic.

12. The future of female fertility preservation

The ovary contains all the eggs that a woman will ever produce within the outer millimetre. Since 1996 specialists have been trying to preserve fertility by freezing and transplanting ovaries or freezing just part of the ovarian tissue from that outside edge for transplantation later on.[7] Primarily this has been for patients with life-impacting medical conditions who did not have time to go through IVF.

The first live birth was recorded in 2004 in Belgium,[8,] and in 2014 the first live birth following the transplantation of ovarian tissue removed during childhood.[9] This raises exciting possibilities for the future and also many ethical questions, too. The first live birth in the UK following the transplantation of stored ovarian tissue was reported in July 2016, the ovarian tissue frozen when the patient was aged twenty-two and stored for eleven years.[10]

During the 2016 annual meeting of the European Society of Human Reproduction and Embryology, results from a pilot study for cancer patients in Oxford included removing ovarian tissue from a two-year-old girl who had cancer, extracting the immature eggs from the tissue and then maturing them prior to vitrification.[11] This eradicates concerns over ovarian tissue containing some of the cancer cells, which could be transferred back when the ovarian tissue is transplanted.

Vitrification has improved the success rates of stored eggs being stable enough to fertilise after warming/thawing and hopefully to go on to produce a pregnancy. But whether in the future women will be exploring preserving their fertility by storing eggs, ovarian tissue or eggs extracted from ovarian tissue remains to be seen . . . exciting times ahead!

References

1. Wallace, W. H. B., Kelsey, T. W., 'Human Ovarian Reserve from Conception to the Menopause', *PloS One*, January 2010, Vol 5 Issue 1.

2. Chen, C., 'Pregnancy after human oocyte cryopreservation', *Lancet*, 1986; 1: 884–886.

3. HFEA 'Fertility Treatment 2014 Trends and Figures', published March 2016.

4. Cao, Y. X., Xing, Q., Li, L., et al., 'Comparison of survival and embryonic development in human oocytes cryopreserved by slow-freezing and vitrification', *Fertility and Sterility*, 2009.

5. The Practice Committees of the American Society for Reproductive Medicine and the Society for Assisted Reproductive Technology, 'Mature Oocyte Cryopreservation: a Guideline', *ASRM*, pp. 37–43, Vol 99, No.1. January 2013.

6. ESHRE Task Force on Ethics and Law, including, W. Dondorp1 et al., *Human Reproduction*. Vol 27, No 5, pp.1231–1237, 2012.

7. Smith, D. 'Fertility Hopes Reborn with Ovary Transplant'. *The Age*, 24 September 1999; R. Highfield. 'Second Fertility Triumph for Fertility Pioneer'; *The Age*, 25 September 1999.

8. Donnez, J., Dolmans, M. M., Demylle, D., et al., 'Livebirth after orthotopic transplantation of cryopreserved ovarian tissue', *Lancet* 2004, 364:1405–1410 [Erratum, *Lancet* 2004;364:2020].

9. Demeestere, I., et al., 'Live birth after autograft of ovarian tissue cryopreserved during childhood', *Human Reproduction* journal, doi:10.1093/humrep/dev128.

10. Carr, R., 'First baby born from frozen ovarian tissue in UK', *BioNews* 860, 18 July 2016.

11. Gilchrist, R., 'Eggs successfully grown from two-year-old cancer patient', *BioNews* 859, 11 July 2016.

CHAPTER 7

Donor (Egg and/or Sperm) Assisted IVF

Laura Spoelstra, former Chief Executive of the National Gamete Donation Trust (now SEED Trust)

1. Introduction by Mollie Graneek, BACP Senior Accredited Counsellor/ Psychotherapist, Harley Street Fertility Clinic

If you are going through fertility treatment and you discover that your best (or only) chance of achieving a family is IVF with donor assistance, your first step should be to undertake infertility counselling.

1.1 What is infertility counselling?

According to the British Infertility Counselling Association, infertility counselling offers patients an opportunity to explore their thoughts, feelings, beliefs and their relationships in order to reach a better understanding of the meaning and implications of any choice of action they may make. Counselling may also offer support to them as they undergo treatment and may help them to accommodate feelings about the outcome of any treatment.

Infertility counselling is a key way in which fertility clinics can be assured that the consent that patients are giving to their treatment choice is truly informed.

1.2 Why is infertility counselling important?

In 1990, the passing of the Human Fertilisation and Embryology Act led to the offer of counselling in licensed assisted conception units being required by law. Although counselling on issues related to infertility was not new, this legislation underlined its importance.

1.3 What to expect from an infertility counselling session

A trained counsellor will provide a secure, confidential environment for you to explore, understand and gain insight into your feelings about your infertility. The counsellor and the patient develop a working relationship and identify the specific needs of you as an individual or a couple. She/he will offer support, empathy and acceptance of painful feelings in a non-judgemental and non-directive manner.

The diagnosis of infertility can often feel like a 'life crisis' and may be difficult to come to terms with. Many patients experience feelings of distress, loss, anxiety, sadness, isolation and frustration – all feelings that can be overwhelming and difficult to deal with. These feelings may affect all your relationships – with partners, relatives, friends and work colleagues. They may affect your self-esteem and sexual relationships.

The counsellor's role is to listen and offer support, helping you to explore ways in which to cope better with your feelings. Often by 'normalising' the feelings that emerge when faced with infertility a certain clarity is gained, enabling patients to embark on the next stage of treatment.

1.4 Is infertility counselling 'mandatory' before IVF with donor assistance?

While infertility counselling is not 'mandatory' prior to IVF with donor assistance, it is strongly encouraged by the HFEA. This is because there are many emotional, practical and legal ramifications that patients must be made aware of. Counselling in the case of donor-assisted IVF also encourages potential parents to consider the important consequences for any future donor-conceived child.

1.5 How to find an infertility counsellor

All UK-licensed fertility clinics are legally required to offer infertility counselling. If you are not satisfied with the standard of counselling offered to you by your clinic,

BICA (British Infertility Counselling Association; www. BICA.net) is a great source of information and counsellor recommendations.

Within this chapter, we'll look at the considerations when going through donation treatment both for yourself and your future child – the ways in which it is different from 'straightforward' IVF, what to think about and what your options are.

Laura Spoelstra explores these topics below.

2. The decision to start donor treatment

If you have gone through fertility treatment with your partner and have achieved a positive outcome – a successful pregnancy – this would in many ways be an 'equal' experience for both of you. In donation-assisted treatment however, at least one of you cannot use your own eggs or sperm, which can result in many mixed and conflicting emotions. The sadness of not being able to have a child that's genetically linked to both of you could change the dynamics in this (until now) shared process. It's possible, and completely normal, that you think differently from each other when it comes to using a donor, but also if the child should know about the donor treatment and when and how to tell your child.

As previously mentioned, donor conception is therefore not right for every couple and it's important that the implications of using a donor in your fertility treatment is talked through carefully. This could be done individually or as a couple, and a specialist counsellor can support both or either of you in this process. 'Implications counselling', as this type of counselling is known, will help you explore the questions that you may not have even thought about.

3. Donation and the law

All IVF and donation treatments carried out by UK-licensed clinics will be registered, licensed and monitored by the legislator, the Human Fertilisation and Embryology Authority (HFEA).

The HFEA holds the data about the donor that is used in your treatment as well as your own information and that of your child.

Donors are asked to provide the following information:

- Name
- Date of birth
- Address
- NHS number
- Ethnic group
- Marital status
- The number of children they already have and their gender
- Physical characteristics like hair colour, skin tone, eye colour, height

- Details of their screening tests and medical history
- A goodwill message to any potential children conceived following their donation
- A personal description

All information will be made available to you at the time of treatment and this will allow you to build up a profile of your donor.

Different information may be available if the donor is not UK based but used a UK clinic. The same legislation applies, however, when it comes to making (identifiable) information available.

When your child reaches the age of sixteen they can apply to the HFEA to receive all the non-identifying information their donor provided when they donated. That is, all the information the donor gave to their clinic, apart from their name, NHS number and last known address. Non-identifying information can also be provided about half-siblings like gender and year of birth. Children aged sixteen or seventeen can also approach the HFEA together if in a relationship with someone else donor-conceived, to confirm they were not conceived with assistance from the same donor.

When your child reaches the age of eighteen they can apply to the HFEA to find all the information their donor provided, including identifying information such as their name, NHS number and last known address. Identifying details about any half-siblings can also be given.

All donors that are used for treatment in UK-licensed

clinics are non-anonymous. That means that at the time of treatment the details of the donor are not known to the parent/s but their full identity can be made known to the donor-conceived once they reach the age of eighteen.

In the case of unregulated sperm donors, it is often confusingly stated that 'clinic donors are anonymous'. What is, however, meant is that at the time of conception the identity of the clinic donor is not known (unless it is a known clinic donor). Donors that go through a UK clinic can become identifiable at the time the offspring turns eighteen.

4. The role of the donor

As part of their treatment all UK sourced donors are counselled to be non-anonymous, or identifiable, donors. At the time of donation all donors must be open to being contacted by the people conceived from their donation once they turn eighteen; there are no exceptions.

Donors donate to enable parents to parent and don't identify as a biological or genetic parent; additionally, the donor is never the legal or social parent and will not be mentioned on the birth certificate when treatment takes place in a UK-licensed clinic. The donor is also not able to seek contact with the donor-conceived without contact being initiated by the donor-conceived themselves.

A donor can find out if a donation has been successful and how many children with their gender and birth year are born from a donation.

A donor can specify the maximum number of families his donations are used for up to the legal maximum of ten. Most donors agree to this maximum.

There is no difference in legislation for an egg donor or a sperm donor. Only the remuneration differs: at the time of writing, £750 for a cycle in egg donation and £35 per visit for a sperm donor.

5. Telling your child about donor conception

In the past, most clinics encouraged prospective parents to forget about their treatment as soon as it was over. It was thought to be unnecessary, and potentially harmful, to tell children about how they were conceived. However, social and professional attitudes have changed, and for the past twenty-five years or so parents have been strongly encouraged to tell their child that they were conceived with the assistance of a donor.

There are many reasons why parents are advised to be open with their child – both from the perspective of a harmonious family life and, most importantly, for the emotional welfare of the donor-conceived child.

These are not just moral and ethical considerations like honesty within the family and being respectful to the donor-conceived. There are other practical and medical reasons why it is advised to tell a person who is conceived with the help of a donor: it helps explain potential differences in looks so the child doesn't worry about it; it also means that there's openness about the medical history – or lack of it. In the case of families with a genetic disorder, it can remove the anxiety about being a carrier. Experts advise making telling about the donor-conception part of their life-story. By taking control of when and how this is being told there is no fear of the information coming out in a crisis situation or via another party.

The ease of access to DNA tests and the relatively low cost of finding out the genetic relationships between family members also mean that the chances of keeping the method of conception a secret are low.

6. How treatment choices impact on your child

Unlike 'normal' IVF, the type of treatment you decide on can have major implications on your child and yourself once the child grows up. People have different considerations, sometimes also fuelled by the available resources. Cost-cutting within the NHS unfortunately does mean that donor treatment is often not funded. It is important that you carefully consider the implications of these options and choices, balancing the best options to start a family with the needs for your future child.

The questions to ask yourself:

- How important is it that you know the donor is medically screened and that the complete medical history has been assessed?

- Is it important what the motives are for the donor?

- Are you sufficiently aware of the importance of telling your child that he or she is donor-conceived and, do you want your child to have the option to find out their genetic roots?

- Is it important to you that there are clear legal boundaries around parenthood?

- How much information do you want from your donor at the time of conception?

- Is it important to know how many half-siblings your child has?

- Can you explain confidently to your child why you made your choice?

7. Support for donor-conception parents

Donor Conception Network is a supportive network of more than 2,000 mainly UK-based families with children conceived with donated sperm, eggs or embryos; those considering or undergoing donor conception procedures; and donor-conceived people. They are inclusive of all families using donor conception, and as children grow up within the Network, they have developed resources and services for them as well as continuing to support parents.

They welcome families who are exploring whether or not openness with their children and others is right for them as well as those who have already made this decision.

For more information go to www.dcnetwork.org.

8. Treatment with donor sperm

Donor sperm is used in different types of fertility treatments or where there is no medical need for treatment (for instance, single woman and same-sex female couples). The type of fertility treatment you will receive depends on your personal circumstances and medical history.

8.1 Intrauterine Insemination (IUI) With Donor Sperm

Before undergoing IUI, it is essential that the fallopian tubes are healthy and open.

This is checked in one of two ways:

- Hysterosalpingo-contrast sonography (HyCoSy): a vaginal ultrasound to check the fallopian tubes for blockages or a hysterosalpingogram, which is an X-ray of the fallopian tubes.

- Laparoscopy: an operation performed under general anaesthetic, where a camera (laparoscope) is inserted through a small incision near your belly button, giving a view of your ovaries, uterus and fallopian tubes. A coloured dye will be injected through your cervix into your uterus and fallopian tubes.

8.2 What happens to the female?

- Unstimulated cycle. If you are having IUI without fertility drugs then you will be inseminated close to when you are due to ovulate. Depending on your clinic, ovulation will be identified by a blood test or urine test.

- Stimulated cycle. Your clinic will provide you with medication to help you produce egg follicles. The clinic will monitor your response to the fertility drugs by transvaginal ultrasounds. When your egg follicles are mature, you will be asked to inject yourself with a trigger shot to release the eggs.

- Before insemination – What happens with the donor sperm? The embryologist will remove the donor sperm from clinic frozen storage and thaw it. It is then clinically washed and the faster-moving sperm will be separated from the slower-moving sperm.

- The insemination. The insemination itself is usually painless and takes just a few minutes. Your clinic will tell you when your insemination will take place, which is usually around 36 hours after you have ovulated. A speculum will be inserted into your vagina to keep the vaginal walls apart. This is similar to a smear test. A small catheter containing the fast-moving sperm will then be inserted through your cervix and into your uterus. Two weeks after the insemination, you can find out if you're pregnant via a blood test at the clinic or a home pregnancy kit.

8.3 IVF (+ICSI) With Donor Sperm

- Suppression or down regulation. This stage of 'suppression' or 'down regulation' can take between two and four weeks. Hormones are taken by daily injection or by daily nasal spray. Sometimes, depending on the medical protocol your clinic decides on, this stage and the next ('stimulation') are merged. Regular blood tests and scans will take place to see if your body is responding to the medication appropriately.

- Stimulation (daily injection for 10–14 days). You take a daily injection for between ten and fourteen days of follicle stimulating hormone (FSH) to stimulate your ovaries to produce egg follicles You will have regular scans and blood tests to see how your body is responding to the medication, including how many egg follicles there are and their sizes.

- HCG trigger injection (one injection 36 hours before egg collection). At the latter stage of the process, the frequency of scans and blood tests will increase to check for the growth and availability of egg follicles. Once it's estimated that release of the follicles is about 36 hours away you will be injected, or inject yourself, with an 'HCG trigger shot', to induce ovulation.

- Egg collection (takes 15–20 minutes). Your eggs will be collected about 36 hours after the 'HCG trigger injection'. This can happen under local or general anaesthetic.

- Sperm preparation. The embryologist will remove the donor sperm from clinic frozen storage and thaw it. It is then clinically washed and the faster-moving sperm will be separated from the slower-moving sperm.

- Introduction of sperm and egg. Once your eggs have been retrieved, the embryologist will prepare and mix them with the donor sperm in the laboratory. Depending on what the clinic has advised, this will either be traditional IVF, where the eggs and sperm are left to meet and fertilise in a Petri dish, or ICSI, where an embryologist will inject single healthy-looking sperm into each of the mature eggs.

- Fertilisation. Embryologists will monitor the fertilisation to embryos and will keep you up to date on their progress.

- Embryo transfer. Depending on the development and number of embryos available, an embryo is prepared for transfer to your uterus. To reduce the risk of a multiple pregnancy, and dependent on your age, the clinic will most likely only transfer one embryo. This needs to be discussed before the actual transfer. A speculum will be inserted into your vagina to keep the vaginal walls apart. This is similar to a smear test. A small catheter containing the embryos will then be inserted through your cervix and into your uterus. Two weeks after the transfer, you can find out if you're pregnant via a blood test at the clinic or a home pregnancy kit.

9. Using a sperm donor

If you need a sperm donor you have various options available to you:

- Treatment via a UK-licensed clinic

- Using a known donor via a UK-licensed clinic

- Going abroad for treatment

- Using unregulated (online) services

During fertility treatment it is normal, of course, to just focus on getting pregnant and not think too much of the impact on yourself and the child later in life. Donor-assisted conception is, however, not the same as 'normal' IVF. By using a donor, there is another person's DNA involved, which will potentially impact on your child's characteristics and health. Not only that, but how the donor conception is dealt with psychologically may well have an impact on the wellbeing of your child, your family and yourself.

It is important that you consider and talk through all the options that are available to you and choose the one that you, and your partner, are most comfortable with now and for the future.

10. Sperm donor treatment via a UK licensed clinic

The recommended route for UK patients is to go via a clinic regulated by the Human Fertilisation and Embryology Authority. The rules around who can be a sperm donor in the UK are strict to protect you as the recipient, your future child and the donor. The reasons for such controls are to provide a safe donation environment for all the parties involved so that everyone's physical and emotional health is protected, and also to offer a clear legal framework around parenthood.

Sperm donors must:

- Be between the ages of eighteen and forty-one

- Be willing to be screened for medical conditions

- Have no known serious medical disability or family history of hereditary disorders

- Know (or be able to find out) their immediate family medical history – children, siblings, parents and grandparents

- Agree to be registered with the HFEA as a donor and be willing to be known to any child born following their donation once the child reaches the age of eighteen

- Not put themselves at risk of sexually transmitted infections (STIs)

- Not knowingly leave out any relevant information

which could affect the health of any children born as a result of their donation

- Be offered implications counselling
- Not receive payment for donating other than compensation for expenses (at the time of writing, up to £35 per clinic visit)

Additionally, sperm donors in the UK can only donate to up to ten families. One of the reasons to limit sperm donations is the risk of accidental consanguinity (intimate relationship between people with a shared ancestor) between donor offspring.

By receiving donated sperm through one of the UK-licensed clinics, your legal parenthood, regardless of your marital status, is as follows:

- You will be the legal parent of any child born following your fertility treatment
- You will be the named parent on your child's birth certificate
- You will be legally, ethically, morally and financially responsible for your child

Your donor will *not*:

- Be the legal parent of your child
- Have any legal obligations to or any rights over your child

- Be named on your child's birth certificate
- Have any financial obligations to support your child

The clinic will try to match the physical characteristics of the donor as much as possible with the male partner. In the case of same-sex couples or single women, it will be matched as much as possible with reasonable wishes.

Unfortunately, there is unequal access to sperm donors in the UK. There are private clinics, mainly in large cities, that will be able to start treatment straight away. However, that is not the case for the majority of clinics and especially not for NHS ones. There's also not a wide range of donors available with ongoing shortages of ethnic-minority donors. Patients requiring sperm from an ethnic minority may therefore have longer waiting times and can be advised to seek a donor within the family or community (for instance when a sister of the future mother becomes an egg donor or the brother of the future father becomes the sperm donor).

The HFEA or the Sperm, Egg and Embryo Donation Trust (www.seed.co.uk) can advise you on clinics that have sperm donors available. The latter, originally the NGDT, is the national body running the National Gamete Donation Services. They support and empower gamete (egg and sperm) and embryo donors and also work with potential recipients, UK-licensed fertility clinics, the media and support organisations to raise awareness of the need for egg, sperm and embryo donors.

11. Using a known donor

You may also decide to use a sperm donor you know, for instance a family member or friend. It is still advisable to go through a UK-licensed clinic to ensure all medical screening takes place and to get clarity on the status around legal parenthood.

Using a known donor who may play some part in your life, and in the life of your child, will have its own set of challenges for all parties involved. 'Implications counselling' is therefore very important to ensure that the expectations of all those involved re: future relationships match.

Although the clinic may waive some of the donor criteria – lower motility or age of the donor – overall the process of using your own known sperm donor will be the same as using another donor in the clinic.

12. Using imported sperm or going abroad

Some clinics import sperm from abroad, mainly the USA and Denmark. While the donors fall under UK legislation and their identifiable details can be made known by the time your child is eighteen, there are some differences to consider and how they might impact on you and your child's physical and emotional wellbeing.

If you're considering going abroad for treatment with donor sperm then it's important to be aware of the following factors and the impact they will have.

- Lack of stringent regulation governing donation in the country of origin (often there is no regulation or it's very different from the HFEA system).
- Donor's screening tests, and personal and family medical history are often not investigated as thoroughly, or at all.
- An absence of counselling for the donor may mean that they are less aware of the implications of their donation.
- An absence of implications counselling for you as recipients might mean that you're affected by issues that may never have crossed your mind.
- There are no international public databases so there's no reliable way of finding out how many children are conceived from the same donor.
- Limits on the number of families a donor can donate to may not exist, meaning that your donor-conceived child could have more than 100 half-siblings.
- An absence of robust recording systems in some countries means that even if sperm donors are willing to be identifiable, the information may not be available when you want it.
- Depending on where your sperm donor is from, your donor-conceived child will likely have very different features and genetic origins from you and your family.

13. Using unregulated services

There are a growing number of women, mainly those in same-sex relationships or single women, who bypass the clinics and use the internet to find a sperm donor. Sperm donors offer their services in various ways: via introduction websites, Facebook pages or via their own websites.

Unregulated services are also often used if people want to co-parent, i.e. want to involve the donor in the parenting role without being in a relationship with the donor.

Using an unregulated sperm donor has its negatives, both for the woman and the child, often not immediately recognised by those considering this route. Although there are many cases where using an unregulated donor works for the parties involved, people need to be mindful of the drawbacks before they embark on this route. Treatment choices now will have a lifelong impact on you and your child and it's important that time and effort is invested in balancing the options available.

13.1 Things to consider when using an unregulated sperm donor

- Legal parenthood could become very complicated. Unless you are married at the time of conception, your donor could legally be the father of your child. This would give him rights and responsibilities that you might not want him to have.

- Donors are not screened for medical conditions.

- There is no information available about any serious medical disability or family history of hereditary disorders.

- Semen is not tested for effectiveness. In other words, the donor may be subfertile or infertile at the time of donation.

- His age and identity are not verified.

- There is no record of any of his donations.

- Although a large number of offspring may seem favourable, confirming his fertility, your child may have to deal with the knowledge of having a large number of half-siblings.

- Your personal safety may be in danger if you meet up for insemination.

- Your donor may have unpleasant motivations for donating in this way.

- You may need fertility treatment for reasons other than needing donor sperm but you won't find out.

14. Egg donation

Unlike sperm donation that could take place outside a clinic – but it's not recommended to do so – egg donation is a treatment that can only take place in a clinic. It is effectively IVF but with another woman's eggs.

Using donated eggs may be an option if:

- You have no ovaries or have had them removed
- You have had cancer treatment which has damaged your ovaries
- You are post-menopausal
- You are producing few or low-quality eggs
- You have repeatedly tried to conceive unsuccessfully using fertility drugs or IVF
- You have had several recurrent miscarriages
- You have a high risk of passing on a serious inherited disorder

When you have to use donated eggs you have the following choices:

- Treatment in a UK clinic with an altruistic donor (the legislator HFEA calls this a 'non-patient donor')
- Treatment in a UK clinic via egg share
- Using a known donor
- Treatment abroad

14.1 Treatment in a UK clinic

Egg donation in UK clinics is regulated by the HFEA. The rules around who can be an egg donor in the UK are very strict to protect you as the recipient, your future child and the donor.

Egg donors must:

- Be between the ages of eighteen and thirty-five
- Be willing to be screened for medical conditions
- Have no known serious medical disability or family history of hereditary disorders
- Know (or be able to find out) their immediate family medical history – children, siblings, parents and grandparents
- Agree to be registered with the Human Fertilisation and Embryology Authority (HFEA) as a donor and at the time of their donation be willing to be known to any child born following their donation once they turn eighteen
- Not knowingly leave out any relevant information that could affect the health of any children born as a result of their donation
- Receive implications counselling
- Not receive payment for donating other than compensation for expenses (at the time of writing, up to £750 per donation cycle)

Additionally, egg donors in the UK can only donate to up to ten families. The reasons for such controls are to provide a safe donation environment for all the parties involved so that everyone's physical and emotional health is protected, and also to offer a clear legal framework around parenthood.

Unfortunately there is unequal access to egg donors in the UK. Some clinics will have a waiting list while others don't. There may be clinics that claim there are no donors at all available in the UK and will immediately refer you to one of their satellite clinics abroad.

Some clinics have egg donors available via egg sharing. This means that another patient who needs IVF treatment for factors not related to egg quality will donate a cycle or part of her cycle of eggs in return for a refund on her own IVF treatment.

By receiving donated eggs through an egg-sharing scheme, all the same HFEA rules and regulations apply, meaning that:

- Your donor must have met the donor criteria

- Your legal parenthood status will be the same as receiving eggs from an altruistic donor

- The information your egg share donor gave to your clinic and the HFEA will be stored and will be available to your future child in the same way as it would be for a non-egg-share donor

- You will be required to have implications counselling

- Your IVF treatment cycle will go ahead as a typical egg-donation cycle, with the exception that around half of your donor's eggs will be kept for her own treatment and the other half will be given to you

As far as possible, the clinic will try to match you with your donor on physical characteristics. In clinics with limited availability this might be very difficult and you may have to wait longer. This is especially the case for ethnic minorities. In these cases, using a known donor, such as a sister or other family member, might be the only option. Known donation is also used by clinics that do not recruit egg donors themselves but offer the egg-donation treatment for patients who bring their own.

Using a known donor who may play some part in your life, and in the life of your child, will have its own set of challenges for all parties involved. Implications counselling is therefore very important to ensure that the expectations of all those involved re: relationships match.

14.2 IVF treatment with egg donation

Once you've been matched with your egg donor, either altruistic or via egg share, the process is the same.

14.3 What happens to you and your egg donor?

- **Synchronising of menstrual cycles between you and your egg donor.** This stage of 'suppression' or 'down regulation' can take between two and four weeks. Hormones are taken by daily injection or by daily nasal spray. Sometimes, depending on the medical protocol your clinic decides on, this stage and the next ('stimulation') is merged. Regular blood tests and transvaginal scans will take place to see if your egg donor's body is responding to the hormone medication appropriately.

- **Stimulation (daily injection for 10–14 days).** Your egg donor will stimulate her ovaries to make egg follicles with a daily injection of follicle-stimulating hormone (FSH) for between ten and fourteen days. Your egg donor will have regular scans and blood tests to see how her body is responding to the medication, including how many egg follicles there are and their sizes. In tandem, you are given medication to prepare your uterus to receive embryos; it does so by thickening the lining. Regular scans will follow the progress, and medication adjustments are made accordingly.

- **HCG trigger injection (one injection 36 hours before egg collection).** At the latter stage of the process, the frequency of scans and blood tests will increase to check for the growth and availability of egg follicles. Once it's estimated that release of the follicles is about 36 hours away, the donor will inject herself, or will be injected with an 'HCG trigger shot' to induce ovulation.

- **Egg collection (takes 15–20 minutes).** Your egg donor's eggs will be collected about 36 hours after the 'HCG trigger injection' at a scheduled procedure. This can happen under local or general anaesthetic. Your donor's eggs may be available fresh or frozen within an egg bank.

- **Sperm preparation.** Sperm, either from the male partner or from a sperm donor, will be prepared by the embryologists. The sperm is clinically washed, separating the faster from the slower moving sperm.

- **Introduction of sperm and egg.** If you are using fresh eggs, once your donor's eggs have been retrieved, the embryologist will prepare and mix them with either your partner's sperm or the donor sperm in the laboratory. Depending on what the clinic has advised, this will either be traditional IVF, where the eggs and sperm are left to meet and fertilise in a Petri dish, or ICSI, where an embryologist will inject single healthy-looking sperm into each of the mature eggs. ICSI is always used if you are using frozen donor eggs, to promote fertilisation.

- **Fertilisation.** Embryologists will monitor the fertilisation to embryos and will keep you up to date on their progress.

- **Embryo transfer.** Depending on the development and number of embryos available, an embryo is prepared for transfer to your uterus. To reduce the risk of a multiple pregnancy, and dependent on your age, the clinic will most likely only transfer one embryo, and freeze any embryos that have developed to blastocyst stage in a healthy state. The number of embryos to transfer needs to be discussed before the actual transfer. A speculum will be inserted into your vagina to keep the vaginal walls apart. This is similar to a smear test. A small catheter containing the embryos will then be inserted through your cervix and into your uterus. Two weeks after the transfer, you can find out if you're pregnant via a blood test at the clinic or a home pregnancy kit.

15. Going abroad for egg donation treatment

If you already know you need egg donation treatment before you have started the clinic path, going abroad directly may be one of your considerations. You don't have to spend too much time on the internet to be made aware of the myriad of options available.

In other cases, you may have started your path with a UK clinic and were advised that your only option was to go abroad for egg donation. There are many clinics that don't recruit donors themselves – and incorrectly claim there are no donors available in the UK – but instead have arrangements with clinics abroad.

Your treatment and monitoring will take place in your clinic in the UK and it's likely that you won't travel abroad until two or three days after your donor's egg collection. Regardless of where the treatment started, if the transfer of embryos into your uterus takes place abroad, the donation will not fall under UK legislation.

The most popular foreign destinations for general IVF

treatment and egg donation are Spain, Cyprus, Greece, Czech Republic, USA as well as many Eastern European countries. This is not surprising because, with the exception of the USA, most treatments are cheaper than in the UK, but the service standards, and most importantly, success rates are good, if not better than in the UK.

The age of the eggs and therefore egg donor has significant impact on the success rates and with, on average, younger donors in those countries than in the UK, it's easy to see why going abroad for egg donation is a popular option.

In any of these foreign destinations the legal framework is profoundly different, which can have significant impact on you and your child later in life. The balancing act of giving yourself the best chance of a family while doing the best for your child in the future is a difficult situation to be in and patients need to be aware of this.

It's important to be aware of the following when you have egg donation abroad:

- There is limited or no regulation around donor conception in most countries.
- Donors' screening tests, and their personal and family medical history are often not investigated as thoroughly as in the UK.
- Donors are anonymous, which means that your child will be unable to find out who the donor is and make connection with her or any of their half-siblings. Though home DNA testing kits are rapidly removing the potential for donors to remain anonymous.
- An absence of counselling for the donor may mean

that they are less aware of the implications of their donation.

- An absence of robust recording systems in some countries means that even if egg donors are willing to be identifiable, the information may not be available when you want it.
- Payment is relatively higher in most countries (in the USA, up to tens of thousands of dollars!), which in some cases suggests exploitation.
- There's no standardisation of non-identifiable information on the donor. In the USA lots of information is made available, but in most other countries, this is often limited to basic physical characteristics and a one-sentence personality description.
- In most EU and Eastern European clinics the donor is chosen by the clinic, rather than by the patient. Depending on where your egg donor is from your donor-conceived child will likely have very different features and genetic origins from you and your family.

16. Support organisations

As already mentioned, the Sperm, Egg and Embryo Donation Trust (www.theseedtrust.org) is the national body (formerly known as the National Gamete Donation Trust) dealing with egg, sperm and embryo donation. They can help you if you have any non-medical questions about your treatment or if you want support in finding your own donor. They operate independently from clinics, so if you want impartial guidance about treatment options do visit the website for more information.

Donor Conception Network (www.dcnetwork.org) can support you and your family through donor conception. They have first-hand experience and can help you with any questions you might have.

BICA (www.bica.net) and the National Fertility Society (www.nationalfertilitysociety.co.uk) are the only professional associations for infertility counsellors and counselling in the UK, seeking to promote the highest standards of counselling for those considering or undergoing fertility investigations and treatment.

CHAPTER 8

Inspirational IVF Stories

Madison's story (sperm donor and IVF)

My career has always been my priority. I'm a lawyer, working for a big investment bank and work long hours in a pretty stressful environment. I do it because, in short, I enjoy it – the buzz, the working under pressure. And the salary, of course.

So, when it came to my fertility, I have to be honest – it really wasn't something I gave much thought to over the years. I was aware that my periods could at times be very painful and I'd often experience abdominal swelling, but I'd just motor on.

And then I reached my late thirties, was single and found myself for the first time thinking about having a child. The main drawback (in addition to my age) was that I wasn't in a long-term relationship and hadn't yet found a life partner with whom I wanted to have children.

Donor treatment

A friend suggested I consider using a sperm donor. At first, the thought appalled me. The idea of having a child with someone I didn't know was very unsettling. Another friend (who'd undergone four cycles of IVF before achieving pregnancy) suggested I investigate the state of my fertility first before considering the donor route. So, I researched a couple of clinics in London and set about getting some routine tests done. The tests showed that my ovarian reserve was pretty good (surprising, given my age, I was told) but they also revealed that I had a condition called endometriosis. I'd never heard of this condition and was quite shocked to discover that I had 'level three' (level four is the worst).

A laparoscopic operation followed, during which much of the endometriosis was lasered away. While the operation was a success, the endometriosis had damaged both of my fallopian tubes so I was told that IVF was my only route to conceiving. Given that use of donor sperm involves the IVF process (to harvest my eggs and fertilise them with the donor sperm), it suddenly became a more 'acceptable' idea to me.

The next step involved researching clinics that offered IVF and a sperm donor programme. I was very keen to understand the legal ramifications of the donor route. I learned the below:

If you're having treatment at a licensed fertility clinic in the UK, the sperm donor will have no legal rights over any children conceived with their sperm. This means:

- The donor has no legal obligation to any children conceived from their donation

- The donor won't be named on the birth certificate

- The donor won't have any rights over how or where the child will be brought up

- The donor won't be required to support the child financially

I was also very keen to know how much (and what sort) of information I would be able to access re the sperm donor. I discovered that sperm donor profiles usually comprise:

- A physical description (height, weight, eye and hair colour)

- The year and country of birth

- Their ethnicity

- Whether they have any children at the time of donation, and if so, how many and their gender

- Their marital status

- Their medical history

- A personal description and goodwill message to any potential children (if they choose to write one at the time of their donation)

Thinking ahead to the future, I wanted to check if my child would be able to contact his or her donor. I found out the following:

- When a donor child reaches sixteen, they'll be able to find out the same information that you can find out about a potential donor at the time of the donation (see list above).

- When they're eighteen they can find out their donor's name, date of birth and last known address and it's up to them if they want to try and get in touch.

Making the decision to go ahead with donor treatment

Typically, perhaps – given my legal background – I became pretty consumed with the practical and legal elements of the donor route. Looking back, I didn't spend a lot of time considering the emotional consequences. When I chose my clinic, I was offered fertility counselling. In fact, it was impressed upon me the importance of meeting with a counsellor. So, I went along for a couple of sessions but didn't particularly enjoy exploring my feelings about the donor route. Instead, I was more interested in others' views on the donor route. My parents were surprisingly positive about it. While they were very proud of all I'd achieved in my career, I think they'd largely given up hope of ever having grandchildren (I'm an only child). Friends' views varied from very encouraging to quiet disbelief that

I was even contemplating the donor route. In fact, one male friend quipped that 'motherhood isn't something you can just buy'. I was floored by that comment and it really upset me.

After months of consideration and despite still having some reservations, I decided that it was 'now or never' and that I was going ahead.

IVF Treatment

I underwent the 'long protocol' hormone treatment. My biggest fear at the time was the hormone injections – and the fact that I'd have to do them myself. I needn't have worried though as the clinic staff were great at training me in how to do it. The epipen was also a great help, as it didn't even look like you were injecting yourself.

Egg collection went well and I was thrilled when I was told that they'd harvested eight eggs (good for my age, apparently). The sperm donation was ready and waiting and on 'fertilisation day' I was expecting good news. When I heard that only two eggs had fertilised I felt crushed. I'd been expecting a better result and it felt very lonely to receive that news, alone in my apartment.

Embryo transfer

After twenty-four hours of feeling quite low, I decided that I had to pick myself up and start rooting for the two embryos that were currently developing in the lab.

When embryo-transfer day came around, I was back to my positive self, feeling determined to succeed. Just before transfer, I was given the opportunity to view the two embryos under a microscope. I was shocked at how emotional I felt when I looked at them. One of the embryos was graded as being of 'better quality' than the other but both were transferred.

The two-week wait

I found the two-week wait very difficult. Up to that point, I'd been preoccupied with the practical stages of IVF treatment. I'd taken two weeks of vacation as I figured being in a stressful work environment wouldn't be helpful. But having two weeks sitting around at home dwelling on it all was tough. I found myself repeatedly reading the donor's profile, obsessing over every detail. I had moments of supreme optimism when I convinced myself the treatment had worked and other darker times when I questioned how rational it was to be having a child with someone I'd never met. It was during those moments that I wished I'd pursued the counselling I'd been offered more thoroughly.

The result

My fertility clinic had advised against using a standard, over-the-counter pregnancy test. Instead, I went for blood tests. The results came through later that day. Bizarrely, the call came through when I was queuing at a supermarket checkout. I could see on my mobile that it was the clinic calling. I knew that the sensible thing would be to let it go through to voicemail and call them back when I left the store. But I couldn't wait to know, so I answered there and then – with a conveyor belt full of groceries and a long queue of impatient shoppers lined up behind me! I wish that I'd waited. As the clinic staff very carefully and kindly told me that I wasn't pregnant, I stood rooted to the spot, phone clutched to my ear, silent tears running down my face.

Taking stock

Having taken two weeks off work, I really couldn't take any more time off. My first day back in the office was tough. I'd been quite open with colleagues about the IVF, so inevitably there were a few people asking me how it'd gone. I made a mental note not to share the fact that I was doing IVF next time around (if there was a next time). My parents suggested I take at least six months before considering trying the donor route again. I took their advice and immersed myself back into the busy day-to-day routine of work.

Deciding to try again

After six months or so, I felt a renewed desire to try again. I returned to the same clinic. The egg-collection process first time around had gone pretty smoothly and I preferred the familiarity of the same clinic rather than starting over elsewhere. I'm not sure why but for some reason I assumed that I'd be able to use the same sperm donor. When I found out that he was no longer participating in the clinic's donor programme, I felt bereft – a real sense of loss. While I'd never met him, I'd grown attached to the few facts that I knew about him. I'd felt somehow that I had a 'silent partner' out there somewhere. Not a partner in the relationship sense but someone who was helping me to achieve my goal of having a child. And now suddenly he was gone. These feelings prompted me to have much more in-depth counselling the second time around.

Counselling

Instead of using the counselling service offered by the clinic, I decided to find a counsellor through BICA (British Infertility Counselling Association). I was keen to pursue counselling away from the clinic setting. Looking back, I think this was because I wanted to air all of my hesitations and concerns regarding the donor route. And I was worried that the clinic counsellor might not 'approve' me for the donor programme if I shared my darkest thoughts. I'm so glad that I did this. The BICA counsellor was fantastic and together we explored all of my thoughts and feelings re the donor route. This meant that by the time I began my second IVF cycle, my mindset was much improved and I was ready to embrace the donor route.

Success

My clinic 'matched me' with a great donor profile. I felt very positive and the second IVF cycle went well. While only six eggs (compared to eight during the first cycle) were harvested, they resulted in four viable embryos. Two of the 'best quality' embryos were transferred and instead of sitting around for the two-week wait, I took a relaxing holiday with my mum.

When results day came around, instead of busying myself after the blood test, I went to a coffee shop over the road from the clinic. I hung out there, reading a book until the results were ready. Instead of taking the results over the phone, I arranged to go back to the clinic and get them in person. This time around, I felt better prepared. If it was a negative result, I was prepared. When I heard the words, 'Congratulations, you're pregnant', I couldn't quite believe it. My bravery to 'go it alone' and pursue the donor route had paid off. I was delighted.

My baby girl was born on a beautiful summer's morning. My mum was with me and friends were quick to descend with flowers and hugs. If I'm totally honest, I did feel some sense of absence (my baby's biological father wasn't with us and never would be), but as I looked upon my beautiful girl's angelic face, I knew I was smitten and that we'd do just fine – just the two of us.

Lessons I learnt

- I found counselling is invaluable. If you think that there's a chance that you'd like children one day – don't do what I did and largely ignore your fertility status until it's too late.

- Even when IVF is going smoothly, it can be a lonely process. If you're going the donor route as a single parent, don't be afraid to ask family and friends for support.

- If you're going the donor route, bear in mind that a previous donor may not be available second time around.

Beth and William's story (unexplained infertility and IVF)

Will and I first started trying for a baby shortly after getting married in 2012. After almost two years of trying but with no success, we asked our GP for some fertility testing. My hormone levels were normal and Will's sperm analysis came back fine too. We felt encouraged by the results, so kept trying for about another six months. By January 2015, we were getting worried. Our GP told us we were experiencing 'unexplained infertility'. Friends of ours, who were undergoing IVF, recommended the private clinic they were using. We asked our GP to refer us.

IUI

At the private fertility clinic, we had various tests done. Again, my hormone levels were normal, my fallopian tubes were clear and I wasn't suffering from conditions such as fibroids, endometriosis or PCOS (polycystic ovarian syndrome). Will's sperm count and quality was fine. The clinic recommended that we try IUI. It's a type of fertility treatment that's less invasive (and cheaper) than IVF. IUI tends to work best for couples who don't have severe fertility problems. IUI works by firstly separating the highest-quality sperm from sperm that's sluggish or non-moving. This sperm is then injected into the womb at the woman's most fertile time of the month. As the sperm are left in the uterus to fertilise the egg naturally, it's a less invasive process than IVF. We were very hopeful that IUI would work for us, but the cycle didn't result in pregnancy. At our follow-up session at the clinic, the consultant suggested we try IUI at least one more time before moving on to IVF. He conceded that IUI tends to be less successful than IVF but as we had no obvious, serious fertility problem he was keen for us to try again. So, we tried IUI again. This time, we got a result. I was pregnant and thrilled! We were warned that the first twelve weeks are vital but felt sure that everything was fine with the pregnancy. We told lots of our friends and even notified our employers. You can imagine our devastation when I miscarried at ten weeks. We were stunned and bewildered.

IVF

We were pretty shaken by losing our baby and couldn't even contemplate any further fertility treatment for a year or so. Eventually, we felt ready to embark on further treatment. Our friends who'd originally recommended the private clinic had since had twins via IVF and we felt encouraged by their fertility journey and success. We decided to return to the same private clinic but instead of IUI, wanted to attempt IVF.

In March 2016, I began the 'long protocol'. This is where IVF is carried out over approximately six weeks and includes two distinct stages. The first stage is 'down-regulation', whereby hormone treatment stops your natural cycle. The second stage is 'egg stimulation' and 'egg collection'. Our friends had warned us about some of the side effects of the hormone treatment (headaches, dizziness, abdominal swelling, etc.) but I seemed to cope well with the IVF drugs.

Egg collection

Post-egg collection, we had eight eggs (one of which was immature and non-viable). The day after egg collection, we received a call from the clinic embryologist telling us that all seven eggs had fertilised. We were over the moon!

Embryo transfer

We were told by our consultant that if we did a 'day 5' transfer, the embryologist would be able to tell at day 5 which embryos had achieved 'blastocyst' stage. Embryos have to achieve blastocyst stage (either inside or outside of the womb) in order to implant and develop into a foetus. Therefore, our chances of success with 'blastocyst' embryos were higher. We agreed to a day 5 transfer. You can imagine our disbelief when, on reaching day 5, we were told that none of our seven embryos had reached blastocysm. There was effectively nothing to transfer. We left the clinic feeling absolutely desolate. We still had to pay for the cycle. It had never occurred to us that an IVF cycle can halt so abruptly at the final stages.

IVF for second time

Despite our devastation, it felt like a different type of grief compared to recovering from the miscarriage. Before, we'd lost a baby. With the first cycle of IVF, we'd fallen at the last hurdle of the process. I felt a renewed vigour and determination to try again. Will took some persuading (IVF is expensive and he was genuinely worried about the pressure it was putting on our finances). Both sets of parents stepped in and said they'd help, taking the financial strain off us. I discovered that I could apply for some unpaid leave from work, so took two months off.

In July 2016, we started IVF for a second time.

Undertaking the 'long protocol' for a second time within the same year helped in terms of 'knowing the ropes'. Again, my body weathered the hormone treatment well. I made the most of my time off work too – taking leisurely walks and generally relaxing and being kind to myself.

Egg collection

Just like the first time around, egg collection went well. I awoke from the anaesthetic to be told that nine eggs had been collected. The next morning, Will and I were on tenterhooks, waiting to hear how many eggs had fertilised. The call from the embryologist came through at 10 a.m. – six had fertilised. While we felt encouraged, we knew better than to 'count our chickens'... having been so crushed by our previous cycle, we pushed for a 'day 3' transfer instead of 'day 5'.

Embryo transfer

Two of our best-quality embryos were transferred on day 3. We were far from knowing the outcome of the cycle but felt a distinct sense of achievement at having got so far.

The two-week wait

The two-week wait felt like the two-month wait. Being off work was great in the sense that I could relax, but it also gave me too much time to dwell on things. Everywhere I went, it seemed as though I saw mothers with babies... the park for a gentle walk – babies. My local coffee shop for a decaff latte – babies. Adverts on TV – babies.

The result

Eventually, results day came. After the blood tests, Will and I went for lunch at a café over the road from the clinic. I think we sat in silence for almost two hours, leafing through newspapers and magazines but not being able to focus sufficiently to read any of them. When the call came though, I suddenly felt too nervous to answer. Will picked up the call. The tears streaming down his face and the enormous grin told me all I needed to know – we were pregnant.

Post twelve weeks

Inevitably, the first twelve weeks were very worrying, but we came through them together and didn't miscarry. We went on to have one beautiful baby (so one of our two embryos successfully implanted).

Would we do IVF again to extend our family in the future? 'One step at a time,' I'd say, but in my heart, I know that I'd travel this journey again.

Lessons we learnt

- Every IVF cycle is unique. Your results can be markedly different from one cycle to another.
- An IVF cycle can suddenly halt at a particular stage. You may not get to complete a full cycle and achieve embryo transfer.
- 'Be kind' to yourself when undergoing IVF. Even the 'small stuff' like taking time to relax can make all the difference to how well you cope with getting through an IVF cycle.

Carla and Maria's story (sperm donor and IVF)

As a same-sex couple wishing to have a family, we knew that fertility treatment would be our only route to having a child with a biological link to at least one of us.

We'd been together for about five years before we discussed having a child. Looking back, I think we both knew that it'd involve invasive treatment and so wanted to feel absolutely secure in the stability of our relationship.

In 2015, at the ages of thirty-five (me) and thirty-seven (Maria), we commenced fertility tests through a private fertility clinic that had been recommended to us.

Fertility testing

The fertility testing was quite extensive. We both had our hormones 'profiled' to measure any hormone imbalance.

My hormones were deemed 'normal' but Maria's were out of balance.

We both had blood tests to find out whether we were ovulating normally. Again, my results came back 'better' than Maria's. At first we thought this was probably because I was the younger partner, but an ultrasound scan of Maria's womb and ovaries revealed that she was suffering from PCOS (polycystic ovarian syndrome).

PCOS

PCOS is a condition in which many small cysts form on the ovary resulting in hormonal imbalances, which can cause infertility. We were told that while PCOS can't be cured, the symptoms can be managed.

Maria was advised to make some lifestyle changes – to lose weight (her body mass index – BMI – was a little high), to exercise more and to eat a healthy, balanced diet. We were told that weight loss of just 5 per cent can lead to significant improvements in BMI.

While Maria felt determined to make the lifestyle changes, we also didn't want to delay motherhood. In some ways, the diagnosis of Maria's PCOS made our decision more straightforward. As the younger partner with no obvious fertility issues, I'd be the one to attempt pregnancy.

IUI

Later during 2015, we made our first attempt at IUI (intrauterine insemination). IUI involves a lab procedure to separate fast-moving sperm from more sluggish or non-moving sperm. For us, this procedure was performed on imported sperm from Scandinavia.

In advance of IUI, I'd had a hysterosalpingogram (an X-ray to check my fallopian tubes) to check that they were open and blockage-free. My fallopian tubes were fine. As I wasn't on fertility drugs, IUI was performed between days 12 and 16 of my natural monthly cycle.

On the day of sperm transfer, I felt very nervous. Maria was incredibly supportive, but it was nerve racking nevertheless. As it turned out, the whole process only took a few minutes and was pretty painless. It's similar to a smear test, but during the process a small catheter is threaded into your womb via your cervix. The best-quality sperm from our donor was then inserted through the catheter.

IUI result

When it came to finding out the results, we asked to do a pregnancy test at home. It felt more personal to find out the result at home together. The pregnancy test was negative, so we ended up going back into the clinic for blood tests anyway.

Inevitably, we were both very disappointed. Bizarrely

though, I also felt some relief. Being the nominated partner for pregnancy, I'd felt a great deal of pressure for the IUI to work. I'd been so caught up in the practicality of the various tests and procedures that I hadn't had a chance to really talk to Maria about how I felt about conceiving a child with donor sperm. It may sound silly but as the donor route was the most practical for us, I hadn't allowed myself to explore my true feelings about it. I just thought that if we wanted a child, then this was what I had to do.

Counselling

When I broached the subject with Maria, she too said she had reservations about the donor route. We decided to get some counselling to work through our hesitations. The private clinic where we'd undergone the IUI had a fantastic in-house counsellor. She encouraged us to face our fears and share our innermost thoughts on the donor route. After a few sessions, we came to the joint conclusion that what we were really struggling with was the fact that we'd never really know our donor. Outside of the profile information provided, we'd never really 'know' him. This revelation led us to consider an option I never thought possible – that we'd approach a 'known' donor – one of our male friends. Now this of course opened up another whole raft of considerations. How would our friend react? If he agreed to donate for IUI, how would it affect our friendship? And how would it affect my relationship with Maria?

IUI with known donor

After taking a good six months to consider our options and have (many) in-depth discussions with our male friend, we decided to go ahead.

IUI the second time around went smoothly. I felt more relaxed than before and we were all hopeful of success. When the results came back negative, we all felt quite bewildered.

The fertility clinic suggested we try IVF but I was wary of the hormone treatment involved. I'd heard some unpleasant stories about the potential side effects.

Mild stimulation IVF

It was suggested we try mild-stimulation IVF. With mild stimulation, I received a lower dose of fertility drugs over a shorter period of time than with conventional IVF. Sadly though, we only got so far through the cycle before having to give up. Only three eggs were collected and none of them went on to fertilise. This left Maria and me feeling very discouraged. Again, I also felt under terrible pressure to achieve pregnancy and Maria felt frustrated that I was having to take on so much of the physical burden of it all. Our friend, while disappointed, remained optimistic. He genuinely wanted to help us achieve our dream of having a family.

IVF

We took a four-month break and then decided that it was 'all or nothing'. We'd try long-protocol IVF once and see where it took us.

We remained with the same private fertility clinic.

Suppressing my natural monthly cycle

The first stage of IVF involved suppressing my natural monthly hormone cycle. I was given a nasal spray to do this and used it for about two weeks. It wasn't too bad an experience but I did suffer some dizziness.

Boosting my egg supply

Once my natural cycle was suppressed, I was given a type of hormone called gonadotrophin. I had to inject myself daily with this for approximately twelve days. The purpose of this hormone was to increase the number of eggs my ovaries produced. Maria helped by preparing the injections for me. I had to do the actual injections myself though, as Maria is quite squeamish about needles. I didn't mind. It felt good to be doing something practical towards our dream of having a baby.

Monitoring progress

The clinic team kept a close eye on my progress. I had regular vaginal ultrasound scans and blood tests.

Approximately 36 hours prior to egg collection, I was given a hormone injection to help mature my eggs.

Egg collection

Egg collection is performed while the patient is under sedation. I was very keen to understand exactly what the procedure would involve. I was told that a hollow needle (attached to an ultrasound probe) is used to collect the eggs from each ovary.

When I came around from the anaesthetic, I had some uncomfortable abdominal cramping. I was told that it's normal to feel a little sore. I also felt very emotional. Eight eggs had been successfully collected.

Post-egg collection I was given pessaries to help prepare the lining of my womb for embryo transfer.

I remember getting home late afternoon post-egg collection. Maria was in a jubilant mood, feeling very positive about the next steps. If I'm honest, I felt groggy (from the anaesthetic) and quite grumpy. After all, I was the one taking the toll of all that the treatment involved.

Egg fertilisation

My eggs were mixed with our friend's donor sperm and cultured in the laboratory for approximately 18 hours. We were told that any eggs that successfully fertilised (embryos) would be grown in the laboratory incubator.

The embryologist then monitors the embryos and selects the best-quality ones for transfer.

Embryo transfer

As I was under the age of forty, we had the choice of transferring one or two embryos.

We chose to transfer two. Transfer occurred on 'day 3' post fertilisation, when the embryos were at 'cleavage stage'.

The transfer process was similar to IUI in that a speculum is inserted. Again, it's similar to having a smear test. A fine tube (catheter) is passed through the cervix, with ultrasound guidance. The embryos were passed down the tube into the womb. It wasn't painful but rather uncomfortable, as you need to have a full bladder when it's done.

The two-week wait

After transfer, we were into the 'two week wait'. Maria wanted us both to take two weeks off work. I was less keen to do so. I was already feeling under increasing pressure for this 'to work' and having two weeks at home with Maria watching my every move and asking me every five minutes how I was feeling wasn't appealing. Instead, we agreed to have a short mini-break and work either side of that. My job is desk-bound, so it's not as though I was busy doing anything overly strenuous.

IVF results

We were thrilled to discover that I was pregnant – but with one baby not two. So, one of the two embryos had gone on to implant and the other had not. I was surprised at how emotional I felt about one of the embryos not having 'made it'. This fact didn't seem to upset Maria. She was wholly focused on the good news that we were expecting a baby. I had to remind myself that I was still experiencing the aftermath of hormone drugs and that the pregnancy hormones were playing havoc with my emotions.

Our baby boy was born during spring 2018. Our friend and sperm donor remains a good friend. We admire the balance he's found with us and our son – interested and engaged but not overbearing or interfering.

We've since considered trying for a second baby but ultimately decided to count our blessings and focus on giving our boy the best upbringing we can.

Lessons we learnt

- Getting a thorough fertility check before commencing IVF is important. Hormone profiling rules out any fertility issues before beginning an IVF cycle.
- We found counselling vital for sperm donor route IVF. We ended up successfully utilising a 'known' sperm donor but it was only through counselling that we were able to reach this united decision together.

Ruth and David's story (unexplained infertility and IVF)

Unexplained infertility

We first started trying for a baby in 2010. At the time I was thirty-six years old and David was thirty-eight. After a year and some tests (arranged via our GP), we were diagnosed with unexplained infertility. We found this very frustrating at the time. Why was it 'unexplained'? Our GP told us that this simply means that no one root cause of our infertility could be identified. We were also told that it can take up to two years to conceive naturally. So we continued trying.

Clomid

After two years of no success, our GP suggested I try Clomid. This is a hormone treatment which is supposed to boost ovulation. After six months, I fell pregnant. We were overjoyed. Alas, our joy was short-lived as I miscarried at eleven weeks.

Miscarriage

The miscarriage hit us hard. I'm ashamed to say I took out a lot of my anger and hurt on David. Our GP suggested counselling, which we eventually undertook as a couple. Looking back, the counselling definitely helped. It gave us a forum in which to air our grief and share our fears of miscarriage happening again in the future. We discussed the option of IVF with our counsellor. While the Clomid had helped me fall pregnant the first time around, I didn't feel like going back on it and waiting however many more months for it to work again. Instead, I wanted to try and take some control over our fertility situation. I felt frustrated with all the 'waiting'.

IVF

In March 2013, we started our first IVF cycle. We were lucky as we lived in a borough where NHS-funded IVF was available to us. We underwent initial testing and it wasn't long before I was immersed in a long-protocol cycle. The staff at the clinic suggested that David might wish to help administer my hormone injections. They said that they could teach him how to do them. David was keen to do this but I didn't want him to. I wanted to handle the injections myself. So, I'd go off and lock myself in the bathroom, effectively taking all the responsibility of the hormone treatment. At first, my body didn't respond as well to the IVF drugs as the clinic had hoped. David and I had a couple of rows over whether I was doing the injections 'properly'. I was furious with him and he backed off completely. The hormone dosages were adjusted by the clinic and my response improved.

Egg collection

Five eggs were collected and we were very hopeful when 'fertilisation day' came around. Disappointingly, only one egg fertilised. It went on to develop into a viable embryo. On embryo-transfer day, we did our best to feel optimistic. Prior to transfer, we asked about the health of the embryo. We were told that there was some 'fragmentation' of the embryo but that there was still a chance of success. I have to admit that my spirits plummeted when I heard the word 'fragmentation'. Didn't that mean the embryo was damaged in some way? I was told that fragmented embryos can result in pregnancy and a healthy baby, so I clung on to that information.

The two-week wait

I work as a flight attendant and booked two weeks' holiday while I waited for the news. It felt like a long two weeks! David was at work and I filled my days taking gentle walks and watching box sets at home. We'd decided not to share the fact that we were undergoing IVF with family or friends. My mum was the only person who knew. As a result, I felt quite lonely. There were only so many times I could keep talking it through with my mum, and David seemed to have run out of positive things to say. At times, I had to remind myself that he was going through this difficult process too and that it must be equally hard on him. It felt like the longest two weeks of my life.

IVF result

On the day of the result, David was due to meet me at the clinic. I was booked in for a blood test that would reveal whether I was pregnant or not. Foolishly, on my way to the clinic, I decided on a whim to buy a pregnancy test. I was so desperate for some element of control that I thought that if I knew the result already, I'd be better prepared. Of course, the worst happened. I'd dashed from the chemist into the nearest coffee shop, done the test in the ladies' loos and then had to sit there for an hour stunned at the negative result. By the time I met David at the clinic that afternoon I was terribly upset. Naturally David was sad too, but I think he also felt very let down that I'd done the pregnancy test without him.

Trying IVF again

We went on to try IVF another two times. The second attempt was also NHS-funded (and at the same clinic as the first attempt). The cycle went reasonably smoothly but ultimately didn't result in pregnancy.

The third (and last) attempt was privately funded. We decided to change fertility clinics for our third IVF attempt. I'd done a great deal of research into fertility clinics and found the HFEA website a really useful source of information. I felt like we needed to 'start over' with a different medical team in a different clinic setting.

Once we'd chosen our clinic, we underwent the same

initial testing as before but greater scrutiny was given to David's sperm results. We were told that David had an issue with the morphology (shape) of his sperm. ICSI was recommended. ICSI is a process whereby sperm are selected for their quality and injected into the egg as opposed to being allowed to penetrate the egg themselves. I really tried to be supportive of David when we received this news. Understandably, he was upset about it and I think it was a bit of blow to his manhood and self-esteem. Looking back, I also felt very annoyed. Not with David but with our previous clinic. Why hadn't they picked this up? Had we undergone two previous IVF cycles with substandard sperm? I felt very let down.

Counselling

We decided to return to counselling – to process our frustration and to support us throughout our third cycle. Again, we'd decided not to tell friends and family (other than my mum) that we were doing IVF. At the time, I felt that this was a way of maintaining some control over what we were going through. I didn't like the idea of having a group of people to 'update' on our progress and then ultimately have to share our result with. As it turned out, this decision to keep it all under wraps had been putting David under increasing emotional pressure. During one of our couples' counselling sessions, he broke down in tears and confessed that he found the secrecy suffocating. Without realising the potential consequences,

I'd selfishly nominated my mum as our only confidante. As a result, I'd always had at least one person (outside of my marriage) to talk to. I'd left David with no one to confide in. I felt terrible when this revelation came out. I was ashamed at how selfish I'd been.

We agreed on two sets of close friends with whom to share our IVF news. Over dinner at home one evening, we told them about our IVF journey so far. They were all so supportive and I could see that David in particular was visibly relieved to be able to finally talk about things with someone other than me.

Our last attempt – success at last!

In October 2015, we went into our third attempt with a renewed sense of optimism. We'd come to terms with our need for ICSI and felt encouraged that it'd improve our chances of success. The clinic had suggested we meet with their in-clinic nutritionist and we'd both embraced a healthy eating plan ninety days prior to starting our third cycle of IVF. Looking back, we felt prepared, positive and, most importantly, united.

Again, I went into a long-protocol cycle. This time around, I let David do some of the injections. Egg collection went well and seven eggs were harvested. ICSI was used and four of the seven eggs fertilised – a record result for us! The embryos were graded by quality and two were transferred. It's hard to explain but I felt markedly different this time around. I felt more calm and optimistic than on any of the previous cycles. David and I had worked through so many pent-up emotions during our counselling that I think we both felt lighter and freer to share our feelings.

We took a very different approach to the two-week wait than before and went on holiday. We didn't do anything too adventurous or strenuous, although I did feel a little paranoid about lying in the sun or getting too hot. We just had a relaxed, lovely time together. And I really tried not to obsess about what the result would be.

On our return to the UK, we literally went directly from the airport to the clinic for the blood tests. I'll never forget our consultant's face when he delivered the happy news – we were pregnant – with twins! We were literally speechless and it took us a good week to fully take in the amazing news.

Our beautiful boys were born in June 2016 – Oliver and Henry.

I am thankful every day that our six-year fertility journey eventually led us to this very happy conclusion. Looking back, the ups and downs also brought David and me closer together.

Lessons we learnt

- Trying to take every step of the IVF journey 'together' was important. As was trying to let David participate in the IVF cycle as much as possible. For example, he learnt how to administer my hormone injections, which took some of the pressure off.

- Trying to be prepared for the amount of 'waiting' involved in fertility treatment. Trying not to put our lives on hold (easier said than done!) when we were going through IVF and trying to look after each other. Our relationship was just as important as the treatment we were going through.

Imogen and Henry's story (surrogacy and IVF)

Our fertility journey is more than ten years long. Henry and I were both twenty-five years old when we married. We knew early on that we wanted children. As we were both so young when we married, we thought that having a family would be straightforward. Sadly, it wasn't.

Repeated miscarriage

Conceiving wasn't an issue for us but holding on to the pregnancy was. We suffered four miscarriages over seven years. During this time, we underwent many fertility tests and investigations to try to understand why this kept happening to us. We eventually discovered that I had a condition called Asherman Syndrome (AS). This condition includes intrauterine adhesions and scarring which can lead to infertility and recurrent miscarriage.

Counselling

We were of course devastated by this news and decided to 'take a year off' from trying to start a family. We needed space and time to absorb the news and consider our options. Our GP suggested we have some couples' counselling with a registered fertility counsellor. We found a really good counsellor through BICA (British Infertility Counselling Association).

Our counsellor firstly helped us to work through our emotions and grief relating to the miscarriages. We'd bottled a lot of these feelings up and I was carrying a great deal of guilt. I'd felt guilty because it was my body that hadn't been able to carry a child full term. I felt as though I'd let myself, the babies and Henry down in the most awful way. It was only when we were encouraged by our counsellor to fully 'feel' those emotions that we could move from 'pain' to 'acceptance'.

After about a year of counselling, we began to feel that we could finally consider other options for achieving a family.

We spent a few months investigating adoption. We continued our counselling and it was through in-depth discussions with our counsellor that we came to the conclusion that adoption probably wasn't the right route for us. We both yearned for a biological connection to any future child we had.

Surrogacy

Through our continued discussions with our counsellor, we came to the conclusion that surrogacy was our best option. Having arrived at this conclusion, we both felt excited and fearful all at the same time. Excited that surrogacy could be the answer to our prayers – a baby who'd be biologically linked to us. And fearful at what the process would entail.

Investigating surrogacy as a route to parenthood

Our counsellor urged us to find out as much as we could before embarking on the surrogacy process.

There are some useful sources of information out there. For example, we found out via Surrogacy UK (www.surrogacyuk.org) that there are two types of surrogacy.

Straight (or traditional) and Host (gestational) surrogacy

Straight surrogacy is the simplest and least-expensive form of surrogacy and is also known as artificial insemination. The surrogate mother uses an insemination kit to become pregnant using the intended father's semen. The baby will therefore be conceived using the surrogate's egg.

We knew that straight surrogacy wasn't for us. We both wanted to be biologically related to our child.

Host surrogacy is when IVF is used, either with the eggs of the intended mother, or with donor eggs. The surrogate mother therefore does not use her own eggs, and is genetically unrelated to the baby. We decided that this was the best route for us.

Researching fertility clinics who offer surrogacy

We took at least six months to research fertility clinics that offered IVF/surrogacy. This is no small undertaking! Again, we found the Surrogacy UK website very useful. It's an organisation that was created by experienced surrogate mothers and reflects their experience of what makes surrogacy successful.

In essence, there are three stages to 'host' surrogacy:

- As the egg donor, I underwent IVF procedures to extract a number of eggs.
- Fertilisation: my eggs were fertilised with Henry's sperm.
- Transfer: the fertilised eggs (embryos) were transferred into the womb of our surrogate mother.

As we were doing a 'fresh' transfer, the monthly cycles of our surrogate and myself had to be synchronised, and this was done using hormone medications.

In cases where embryos have been frozen already and the defrosted embryos are being transferred, the surrogate takes hormone medications to 'ready' her womb lining.

We learned that all clinics vary in practice, but below (courtesy of www.surrogacyuk.org) is an example of a cycle where the intended mother is the egg donor, and there is a fresh egg transfer.

When	What happens
Day two or day twenty-one of the surrogate mother's menstrual cycle	The surrogate mother's natural hormones are 'down regulated' with hormone medication.
Twelve days later	Down regulation of the surrogate mother is confirmed by a vaginal ultrasound scan.
After this	The egg donor starts daily injections to boost egg production. The surrogate mother starts daily oestrogen tablets to build up the lining of her womb.
When both the surrogate mother and the egg donor are ready – usually twelve to fourteen days after the step above	All suitable eggs are collected and fertilised with the father's sperm.
Two to five days later	Up to two embryos are placed into the uterus of the surrogate mother. Any remaining embryos that are of suitable quality will be frozen for use, if needed, in future attempts.
Ten to fourteen days later	Pregnancy may be confirmed.

When	What happens
Six weeks after a positive test result	Viability scan takes place. The clinic will inform your GP and the pregnancy will then be treated as any other pregnancy, with care being given by the surrogate mother's local NHS team.
If the treatment has been unsuccessful	The surrogate will be advised to stop all medication and a heavier than normal period will start a few days later. You should also be offered a follow-up consultation where further options will be discussed. If all parties involved decide to try another transfer, you will need to wait for at least another month before treatment can continue, and most clinics suggest two periods occur after IVF before trying again.

For couples who are not in the position where they can use their own eggs and/or sperm, there are other options such as 'host surrogacy' with donor eggs and/or sperm.

We were very lucky. Our first host surrogacy attempt worked. Our surrogate became pregnant and carried our son successfully to full term.

I can't begin to explain the gratitude we feel towards our surrogate. We deliberately chose a surrogate who had been through the process successfully at least once before. We were careful to be sensitive to her needs, but I have to admit it was very difficult not calling her every day to ask how she was feeling! We managed to find a balance, however, and she will always be very important to us.

Our son, Ryan, is now three years old and we've begun discussions with our surrogate regarding a second child. Whatever the future holds, we feel grateful every day for our beautiful boy – and for our amazing surrogate, without whom parenthood wouldn't have been possible for us.

Lessons we learnt

- A fertility journey is exactly that – a journey. We found it best to take it a step at a time, allowing ourselves time to process each stage of our journey, taking time to grieve and 'process' each previous stage before moving on to the next.
- Being open to alternative paths to parenthood was essential for us. Many of us have preconceived ideas of how we wish to achieve our families. These preconceived ideas can get in the way of other options. Researching routes to parenthood was also essential for us. Knowledge is power.
- We researched, researched, and researched, giving us the most up-to-date information on surrogacy. Investigating support organisations was another essential for us. Researching and visiting a selection of fertility clinics that offer IVF/surrogacy before selecting the one we felt most comfortable with.
- We found counselling to be a vital part of the

surrogacy route to parenthood. Implications counselling helped us to address our true feelings about the process. It also helped us to plan how/what we are going to tell our child about the way in which he was conceived.

Index